Counseling for Hearing Aid Fittings

Edited By

Robert W. Sweetow, Ph.D.

Director of Audiology
Clinical Professor of Otolaryngology
University of California, San Francisco
San Francisco, California

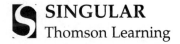

SINGULAR
Thomson Learning

Africa • Australia • Canada • Denmark • Japan • Mexico • New Zealand • Philippines
Puerto Rico • Singapore • Spain • United Kingdom • United States

NOTICE TO THE READER

COPYRIGHT © 1999
Singular Publishing Group is a division of Thomson Learning. The Thomson Learning logo is a registered trademark used herein under license.

Printed in the United States of America
2 3 4 5 6 7 8 9 10 XXX 05 04 03 02 01 00

For more information, contact Singular Publishing Group, 401 West "A" Street, Suite 325 San Diego, CA 92101-7904; or find us on the World Wide Web at http://www.singpub.com

Library of Congress Cataloging-in-Publication Data:

Counseling for hearing aid fittings / edited by Robert W. Sweetow.
    p. cm. — (A singular audiology textbook)
    Includes bibliographical references and index.
    ISBN 1-56593-937-9 (alk. paper : soft cover)
    1. Hearing aids —Fitting.   2. Hearing impaired—Counseling of.
3. Audiology.   I. Sweetow, Robert W.   II. Series: A Singular audiology text.
    [DNLM: 1. Hearing Aids.   2. Audiology.   3. Counseling—methods.
WV274 C855 1999]
RF300.C68   1999
617.8'9—dc21
DNLM/DLC
for Library of Congress   98-32456
                                                              CIP

C

Contents

F

Foreword

The audiologist's understanding of and willingness to address the impact of the hearing impairment on each patient's daily life is a critical component in the success of every hearing aid fitting. Counseling (an essential ingredient of audiologic rehabilitation) is the golden thread that integrates all of our professional interactions with patients and reminds us to address their communication needs as well as provide them with devices. The chapters in this book serve to place the hearing aid fitting back into the context of communication effectiveness.

Robert Sweetow has assembled a group of successful clinicians to contribute chapters to this book. They present the reader with practical information based on clinical experience to help develop skills and confidence in this essential and critical aspect of audiologic practice. The material presented in this book has been selected and brought together to teach and inspire hearing health care givers. The ideas shared skillfully weave together the essential thoughts of audiology. In a sense, Dr. Sweetow is helping to remind us of the roots of audiology (i.e., the rehabilitative needs of Veterans returning from World War II with hearing impairment).

This book takes us through the process of providing good and thorough hearing health care. As the intake case history interview is performed, the audiologist is considering the rehabilitation needs of the patient. During the assessment, implications for future informational counseling are being considered. In the hearing aid selection process, the audiologist provides information and options that are selected to address the demands of each patient's lifestyle. The initial fitting is completed with the patient's individual needs and communication concerns in mind. Information is provided in a manner and at a pace that the patient and significant others can absorb. Woven through all of these interactions is the focus on reducing the communication disorder caused by the hearing loss. This focus allows the audiologist to introduce instruments (whether hearing aids or assistive devices) in the context of rehabilitation rather than sell products designed to "cure" hearing loss. Presenting the hearing aid fitting as an integrated part of the tapestry of individual counseling and rehabilitative needs is more effective than simply dispensing a device.

Robert Sweetow's technical expertise is well known. His understanding of the intricacies of rapidly evolving hearing aid technologies has been demonstrated by his numerous articles, chapters, and presentations. A possibly less well known fact about this audiologist is his firm belief that technical expertise is necessary, but not sufficient, to ensure successful hearing aid adjustment. This belief that counseling the hearing aid user is an equally important component of the hearing aid fitting process is evident in this book.

In responding to questions about his motivation to provide this counseling book, Dr. Sweetow described a situation that may be familiar to the reader. Student audiologists often spend 90% of the time scheduled for a hearing aid fitting appointment "nailing the target," thus leaving only 5 or 10 minutes to counsel the patient. These students are not alone. Many audiologists have stated that they are more comfortable with the technical aspects of hearing aid fitting because their training programs have not offered adequate experience in counseling and audiologic rehabilitation for them to feel confident. This book addresses this issue and provides the information and strategies to help the audiologist develop these skills. We heartily agree with its purpose.

Judy E. Abrahamson, M.A.
Hear Again
Austin, TX

Donna S. Wayner, Ph.D.
The Hearing Center at Albany Medical Center
Albany, N.Y.

Preface

Among the strengths of a multi-authored book is the presentation of diverse opinions. However, there is always the danger of mixing too many styles, thus yielding a publication filled with disparate terminology and formats. Therefore, to make this book as readable, useful, and clinically applicable as possible, the following guidelines were established.

Selection of Authors

The purpose of this book is to provide a practical guide for counseling strategies. Therefore, professionals who have had years of proven success with hearing aid fittings in the "real world" wrote each chapter. The goal was not to put together a compendium of theoretical or research treatises. Instead, it was to share clinical techniques and strategies that have proven to be beneficial.

Chapter Order

Successful fitting of hearing aids is a process, not a single event. It begins with the initial case history and diagnostic testing and does not end until after the patient has received proper orientation and long-term rehabilitation training. In this book, chapters are generally positioned in chronological order according to the chain of events that occurs during the hearing aid process.

Transition Pages

A transition page written by the Editor can be found between chapters. The purpose of the transition page is to link the concepts from the previous chapter to those in the following chapter. Also, because different authors wrote each of the chapters, and much of their material is based on the personal experiences and biases of the authors, the transition pages will acknowledge controversial views and differences of opinions.

Terminology

Rather than impeding the flow of reading with confusing gender terminology such as he/she or s/he, patients are always referred to in the male gender, and professionals are always referred to in the female gender. This is in no way meant to infer that most hearing health care professionals are women or most patients who are hearing impaired are men. It simply makes for an easier read!

The term "hearing health care professional" is a rather wordy one. The majority of the readers of this book are likely to be audiologists, but it must be recognized that there are also many traditional hearing aid dispensers who provide excellent services to the hearing impaired. Therefore, the labels "provider," "dispenser," "clinician," "specialist," and "therapist" refer to either audiologists or hearing aid dispensers. Recipients of professional services are called patients (the customary label in terms of a medical model) or clients (the customary label in terms of a sales approach or client-centered therapy).The selected terminology was chosen by the chapter author.

References and Appendixes

References have been used sparingly on purpose in order to maintain the flow of reading material. The book is designed to be a hands-on guide. Whenever possible, handout materials, forms, and scales are reprinted in their entirety as Appendixes at the ends of chapters. You are encouraged to copy these forms, or download them from the enclosed IBM compatible diskette for immediate incorporation into your clinical practice. In addition, Chapters 7, 8, and 9 contain extensive materials in their Appendixes that can prepare clinicians for hearing aid orientation and aural rehabilitation classes, as well as provide parents of children who are hearing impaired with essential support materials and lists of resources, organizations, educational options, and laws governing amplification and education.

Dialogue Boxes

In the bordered and shaded boxes found in most chapters are sample dialogues or materials that are suitable for easy conversion to patient handouts or brochures.

"Wow" Effect

As Editor, one of my main objectives was to experience a "wow" effect from each chapter. In other words, I only considered a chapter worthy of inclusion if at some point during my reading I said, "Wow, what a good idea."

A

Acknowledgments

It took a lot of people to help put together this book. I would like to first acknowledge the chapter authors, each of whom gave up considerable time from their busy clinical practices to share some of their "secrets to success." Next, my sincere thanks go to Jeff Danhauer, whose editorial suggestions were invaluable. I would like to recognize and state a newly found respect for all the pioneers of aural rehabilitation who sometimes get forgotten in the mountain of technical research we are forced to ingest. One of the most difficult parts of this endeavor was trying to emphasize the professional, ethical aspects of sales, in view of the historically altruistic position in which we audiologists like to see ourselves. I would like to thank my brother, Alan, for his numerous sales and business "tips." If I didn't know he was a car dealer, I would probably buy my next set of hearing aids from him. Last, but not least, there are two groups of people to whom I am most indebted. The Audiology staff members at UCSF have been a wonderful inspiration for me both professionally and personally. In the past year, they have pinch hit for me on numerous occasions and have given me an abundance of extremely helpful editorial suggestions. They are all wonderful counselors, by the way. The individuals who have been most affected, however, during this past year of intense writing and editing are the ones who stand by me always, my wife Linda, and my daughters Kimberley and Rachel. Without their support and love, this project would never have been completed.

RS

Contributors

Marlene Bevan, Ph.D.
AudiCare Hearing Centers
Traverse, Michigan

Becky Bingea, M.A.
University of California,
   San Francisco
San Francisco, California

Joyce Johnson, M.A.
Kenwood Hearing Center
Toledo, Ohio

Rosemary Faucette
Innerwise Consulting
Fayetteville, Arkansas

Kathy Matonak, M.A.
Kaiser Hospital
Santa Rosa, California

Elaine Mormer, M.A.
University of Pittsburgh
Pittsburgh, Pennsylvania

Lori Pakulski, Ph.D.
Eastern Michigan University
Ypsilanti, Michigan

Catherine Palmer, Ph.D.
University of Pittsburgh
Pittsburgh, Pennsylvania

Rennae Pickert, M.S.
Sound Hearing Solutions
Dallas, Texas

Carole W. Shelton, M.A.
Fayetteville, Arkansas

Helena Solodar, M.S.
Audiological Consultants
   of Atlanta
Atlanta, Georgia

Robert W. Sweetow, Ph.D.
University of California,
   San Francisco
San Francisco, California

Robert M. Traynor, Ed.D.
Audiological Associates
Greeley, Colorado

Counseling: The Secret to Successful Hearing Aid Fittings

■ Robert W. Sweetow, Ph.D. ■

This is a book about listening. It is about learning to listen and teaching others to listen. As hearing health care professionals, our primary objective is to supply individuals who are hearing impaired with the tools to hear. Technology has bestowed new and advanced devices on professionals to achieve this goal. But as the old saying goes, "You can lead a horse to water, but you can't make him drink." Statistics suggest that despite technological improvements, we have neither increased our market penetration, nor significantly enhanced satisfaction among those who have "taken the plunge" and purchased hearing aids.

Additionally perplexing is the continuing double-digit return-for-credit rates and the wide disparity of return rates among dispensing professionals. There is no evidence to suggest that lower return-for-credit rates equate with greater mastery of fitting amplification, greater patient satisfaction, or greater patient benefit. However, one cannot question the reality that if we do not get patients to wear hearing aids, we are not providing them with the maximum opportunity to enhance their hearing.

2 ■ COUNSELING FOR HEARING AID FITTINGS

If we accept the notions that (1) our ultimate objective is to help people hear better; (2) the primary means to that end is to get patients to purchase and wear hearing aids; and (3) market penetration continues to hover around 20%, then we need to acknowledge that we are doing something wrong. We need to ascertain what that something is, and how we might correct it. To answer these questions, we must examine the factors that account for the success or failure of a hearing aid fitting. Among the most important are:

■ the product
■ selection and fitting procedures
■ attributes of the professional
■ characteristics of the patient
■ expectations of the patient

In recent years, technological improvements such as digital signal processing, multiple microphone arrays, and advanced compression have provided patients who are hearing impaired with higher fidelity signals than ever before. In addition, we now have a variety of non-linear prescriptive fitting techniques that presumably add to the fitter's ability to ensure audibility (although there are no data to verify that any of these prescriptive approaches correlate with greater patient satisfaction). The attributes of the professional have presumably remained relatively constant over the years, with the exception that, hopefully, the knowledge base has increased. The characteristics of the patient, aside from the status of his hearing, include such variables as motivation, attitude, and patience. Although the stigma of wearing hearing aids unfortunately persists, we maintain hope that with the aging of the baby boomers, this disposition may lessen. The expectations of today's consumers who are hearing impaired may be at an all time high as a result of the media hype surrounding new developments. In fact, all the marketing hype on high-tech hearing aids shifts patients' perceived responsibility away from themselves and onto the hearing aids and the dispensers. So, if we assume that the products and selection and fitting procedures have improved, yet ultimate satisfaction and market penetration have not, then it stands to reason that either the characteristics of the professional and/or the patient have diminished, or the expectations of the patient have risen to an unrealistic level.

Is it possible that our attraction to high technology and the time restrictions dictated by managed care have combined to create an environment in which an inordinate amount of time is spent programming and matching prescriptive targets, at the expense of time spent counseling and teaching patients how to listen? Bear in mind that audiology began as a rehabilitation profession. Are we so seduced by fancy computer programming and prescriptive formulas that we have abdicated our duty to listen to the needs of patients and convey information in a manner that will allow them to have realistic expectations and long-term achievements? Have we become so enamored with computers and high technology that we have lost sight of our objective?

It is the contention of this author that we have either forgotten, ignored, or never learned the fine art of counseling. Moreover, it is this often overlooked element in the total rehabilitation equation that may just be the most important component of all. We have elected to be in a communication profession, yet we seem to be failing to communicate the significance of hearing aid use as a vital strategy. Why is that? Certainly part of the answer lies in the fact that in most graduate level curriculums, audiologists receive little training in counseling techniques. We have had to learn these skills by using our common sense, watching the behavior of other audiologists, and reading the patient's reactions to what we say; kind of a "learn as you go approach."

WHAT IS COUNSELING?

Counseling is the gathering of data through careful listening, the conveying of information, and the making of adjustments in one's strategies based on that knowledge. It is generally a lot simpler to present information than it is to obtain it. Humans tend to have a harder time listening than they do speaking. Perhaps that is the reason why we have two ears but only one mouth! We expect our hearing aid-wearing patients to listen (even without being taught to do so), yet many of us have not mastered this critical skill.

The purpose of this book is to provide strategies to help the hearing health care professional become a better counselor and, thus, perform successful hearing aid fittings. Most of us are in this profession because we care about people and want to make a positive impact on peoples' lives (goodness knows, it can't be the money!). We can have all the state-of-the-art equipment, all the knowledge in the world, and all the sophisticated products at our fingertips, but if we cannot effectively interface amplification with enhanced communication strategies or convey information in a manner that patients can understand and relate to, we have failed in our jobs.

COUNSELING TECHNIQUES

There are two main approaches to counseling: professional-centered and client-centered. In the *professional-centered approach:*

■ the professional asks questions
■ the professional is in control
■ the professional's role is to help diagnose, reach conclusions, and report
■ the professional makes decisions regarding the needs of the client
■ the professional is responsible for all decisions

The counselor using this approach in a hearing aid consultation would tell the patient, "There are a lot of options but by listening to your statements, I have ruled out certain things and have reached a decision as to which hearing aids you should obtain." There are many patients who, given the choice, will elect for you to take a professional-centered approach. These individuals believe they are coming to you for information and answers. They merely want to be told what to do, and they will comply. One major problem with this approach, though, is that if you make all the decisions and the hearing aids fail to satisfy the patient, then it is likely that the patient will accept no responsibility, and the blame will fall squarely on your shoulders.

The *client-centered approach* is characterized by:

■ empathetic listening
■ unconditional positive regard
■ counselor congruence
■ listening with concern

With this approach, the counselor's task is to determine the client's needs, desires, and fears through the use of open-ended questions. The client is the center of the counseling effort, not the professional. The professional serves as a facilitator, rather than as a director. The counselor should not act as someone who has all the answers (because she certainly doesn't, and because clients don't trust anyone who pretends to be omnipotent). Client-centered counseling may be proportional to the number of words not spoken by the counselor. Knowledge is imparted based on the client's needs, not the professional's. The client is held responsible for decisions and outcomes. The client is empowered to make decisions. In fact, your goal as the counselor should be to encourage the client to make decisions and, if not, to get the client to ask you to make the decision. These concepts and a structured approach called Directed Discovery are described in detail by Carole Shelton and Rosemary Faucette in Chapter 2.

LEARNING TO LISTEN

The first rule of counseling is listening! This is how information is gathered. The foundation of all counseling is in inviting reaction and paying careful attention to verbal and nonverbal responses. The counselor must read the patient's emotional state and deal with emotions (e.g., grief, denial, depression, and anger). Asking open-ended questions and using mirroring techniques (as described in Chapter 2) will encourage patients to share their feelings. The patients' comments and reactions should dictate the professional's flow of counseling. The course of a session can be irreparably damaged if the patient believes you are not really listening to him. To demonstrate your attentiveness (which is the foundation of trust), remember a few simple guidelines:

- while taking notes, don't lose contact with the patient
- don't ask questions the patient has already answered
- if you ask a predetermined list of questions, there will undoubtedly be some repetition in either the questions or the answers
- use a waiting room questionnaire and/or expectation survey
- let the patient know you are truly listening by occasionally rephrasing his statements

The term "rephrasing" was purposely used in the above comment rather than "reflection." Simple reflection of the patient's remarks may fail because they may not convey underlying feelings or attitudes. For example, compare these two reactions to the remark: "I can't hear my wife when she talks from the other room."

Reaction 1: "So you're having trouble hearing your wife, especially when she's not in the same room." (To which the patient is likely to think, "Duh, I just said that!")

Reaction 2: "I assume that it's important for you to hear your wife, and the fact that you're not is creating some uneasiness between the two of you." (This remark will invite further comments from the patient regarding the effect that his hearing loss is exerting on family dynamics.)

The purpose of listening is not to offer advice. Rather, show your interest, allow the patient to express himself in a non-threatening manner, and try to understand the feelings underlying the patient's statements. Keep in mind, however, that not all patients are willing or able to express their feelings in a clear, concise manner. In these circumstances, it can be helpful to utilize some of the following counseling techniques:

- Plead naiveté. (Like television's famous detective, Lt. Columbo, play stupid to get the patient to define his statements better.)
- Guide the patient's discovery. ("Then what?" "What would happen if?" "What does that mean?").
- Describe the feelings that other patients have expressed and ask the patient if he feels similarly.
- Reverse roles. Ask the patient to assume the role of a spouse or friend, while you assume the role of the individual who is hearing impaired.

In addition to guided discovery (use of a questioning format to assist patients in reaching conclusions) many of the methods employed by cognitive therapists can be used with patients who are hearing impaired. For example:

- Encourage the patient throughout the session to be active in the process.
- Use excellent listening and empathetic skills.
- Recognize the patient's internal reality with empathy, not sympathy.
- Display high levels of warmth, concern, confidence, and genuineness.
- Be confident and professional.
- Work with the patient to determine prioritized target goals.
- Continually check with the patient to determine his understanding of strategies and techniques being employed.
- Focus on key thoughts, and help the patient recognize dysfunctional thinking that might prevent successful use of hearing aids.

WHAT DO OUR PATIENTS WANT FROM US?

Patients want to have faith in three things about professionals:

1. that we know what we are talking about
2. that we care about them as individuals
3. that we have their best interest at heart and will act upon that

We must establish ourselves as having the knowledge, the desire, and the ability to help the patient effect a desired change. Before we can offer advice that is regarded as having great value we, however, must convince the individual of our desire to be part of the solution. We must make the individual believe that we not only can help provide the answer to his hearing problem, but that we are emotionally vested in providing it to him ... In short, that we care! Personalize the circumstances (e.g., "If I were treating my mother, I would suggest that she . . .") and liberal, but not pretentious, use of compliments (e.g., "Not everyone has the ability to understand what I'm saying, so it's a pleasure to work with you") help put the patient at ease. Demonstrate your honesty and genuine concern (e.g., "If you're only going to wear your hearing aids in limited situations, you probably don't need to spend a lot of money on the highest tech devices," which is analogous to saying, "If you're only going to use your car to drive from your house to the corner grocery store, then you don't need a Ferrari.").

Excluding restrictive mandates from managed care organizations, patients have a choice of specialists from whom to obtain their hearing care. Many patients are aware that the majority of dispensers and audiologists have access to nearly all of the models of hearing aids commercially available. Because the same hearing aids can be obtained from most dispensers, it is important to persuade patients that *you* are the difference! Convince patients that the products you are dispensing are superior and worthy of their cost because your products consist not merely of hearing aids but rather of the process of improving their quality of life. Educate the patient that the appropriate combinations of hearing aids, assistive listening devices, aural (or audiologic; see Chapter 8) rehabilitation, and counseling can keep individuals who are hearing impaired from allowing their quality of life to deteriorate by becoming socially isolated, withdrawn, and dependent on others.

INFLUENCE OF PERSONALITY FACTORS

There can be no "cookbook" approach to counseling patients because counseling strategies should constantly be modified as a function of the responses of the patient and of the particular circumstances involved. Two patients with identical hearing loss may need to be treated differently, not only because of their diverse acoustic demands, but also because of their dissimilar personalities. Learning how to glean personality characteristics from patients will help you adjust your counseling strategies. For example, patients who are outgoing, verbally communicative, and highly social may be dealt with quite differently than patients who are shy and socially withdrawn. By understanding the patient's personality, you may be able to determine whether a patient who says "I'm not sure I need hearing aids" means "They're too expensive," "They're too big," "My brother-in-law hates his hearing aids," "Everyone else mumbles," or "I'm going to look like an old man." Counseling strategies, particularly when it becomes time to convey information, may need to be modified depending on whether the particular patient with whom you are working is a visual learner, an auditory learner, or a tactile learner. In addition, understanding your own personality factors will help you develop the counseling style with which you are most comfortable. In Chapter 3, Robert Traynor discusses one approach to characterize personality types and suggests ways of modifying your counseling strategies based on that information.

CONVEYING INFORMATION TO PATIENTS

If you think professionals are sometimes overwhelmed by all the new technological information crossing our desks each day, think how patients must feel when faced with hearsay, media hype, and the prospect of making decisions regarding purchases of several thousand dollars. As technology evolves, we must constantly strive for new ways to educate in a manner that will neither overpower, nor insult, a patient's intelligence. Given the wide range of sophistication among patients (and dispensers and audiologists, as well), it is not an easy task to gauge the depth of education you should offer. In Chapter 4, Lori Pakulski considers procedures for conveying understandable information to laypersons. Contained in that chapter are numerous examples of explanations that can easily be adapted into handouts for take-home materials and brochures or newsletters.

MATCHING TECHNOLOGY TO THE NEEDS OF THE PATIENT

Physicians use a sequence of questions ordered on the basis of previous answers to arrive at a diagnosis. Similarly, audiologists and hearing aid dispensers must carefully select the proper questions and sequence them based on the patient's verbal and nonverbal responses to arrive at a decision regarding which model of hearing aids should be prescribed. The needs assessment of a patient is a vital component that extends beyond the clinical test battery. Knowing which questions to ask and how to respond to patients' answers will assist the hearing aid fitter in ascertaining which features are necessary and desirable for a given patient.

Prognosis for medical conditions is determined both by the physical examination and by counseling interaction. Similarly, for hearing aids, the correct and relevant clinical battery coupled with establishment of goals and guidance of realistic expectations, usage, and listening skills combine to determine the prognosis for successful adjustment to amplification.

Surgeons employ techniques with which they are familiar. Part of the decision regarding which specific model to select for a patient must be based on the dispenser's mastery of the product. The numerous options available mandate that the dispenser maintains an unparalleled knowledge base and continuing education. In Chapter 5, Marlene Bevan describes the thinking processes that the professional must go through to determine the best product match for patients.

THE ROLE OF SELLING IN OUR PROFESSION

Audiologist David Pascoe (1980) said, "although it is true that more detection of a sound does not ensure its recognition; it is even more true that without detection the probabilities of current identification are greatly diminished." Likewise, it is fair to say that while it is true that wearing hearing aids does not assure good listening skills, it is even more true that the hearing impaired listener who does *not* wear hearing aids is even more likely to not have the ability to listen well.

The word "sale" may have four letters in it, but it is not a dirty word. Some readers of the material contained within this book might believe it is beneath our profession to emphasize the importance of selling hearing aids. But the truth is that the emphasis is not simply on selling hearing aids. It is on selling the process of hearing, and hearing aids are a means to that end. Without the eventual sale of hearing aids, we cannot sell the process of hearing. In Chapter 6, Rennae Pickert considers "How to Sell Hearing Professionally."

Selling and counseling cannot be separated. To sell, we must present an image that instills confidence. To sell, we must recognize the considerable resistance patients have to wearing hearing aids. Practically no one wants to wear hearing aids, and certainly no one wants to spend money or waste time solving a problem unless he perceives that one exists. As mentioned in nearly every chapter, denial of the problem is extremely common. How often do we hear our patients say, "I am only here because my wife thinks I can't hear," or "I can't believe how everyone around me mumbles." Denial of a hearing problem occurs for three main reasons:

- the hearing loss has occurred slowly, so day-to-day changes are minimal
- the patient harbors anger about the origin of the loss
- the patient associates hearing loss with aging (hearing may be the standard that determines whether one considers himself young or old).

Furthermore, to sell, we must recognize that opposition to wearing hearing aids also arises for three main reasons:

- hearsay ("My uncle bought hearing aids and they just sit in his drawer.")
- cost ("Why do these things cost so darned much?")
- stigma ("People will think I'm handicapped.")

Unless this opposition is recognized and addressed, the probability of failure is increased.

Hearing aids are among the few products in the United States that are regulated by laws stating mandatory trial periods. To some extent, such consumer protection laws are necessary to protect patients from unscrupulous sales practices. On the other hand, when we say, "Just try it." we are giving the patient permission to fail. The "30-day trial period" must be applied in a manner that doesn't encourage patients to shirk their responsibility and increase the likelihood of nonsuccess. But if patients don't succeed with hearing aids, we must then direct our attention to alternative rehabilitative approaches in order to provide the patient with opportunities for communication enhancement and to prepare them for the possibility of future attempts with amplification.

Consumers (perhaps unknowingly) are aware that value equals benefit divided by cost. When questioned about the high cost of hearing aids, I often remind the patient (following a thorough discussion of the wide range of benefits that can accrue from improved hearing) that a pair of $5,000 hearing aids having a life expectancy of 5 years equate to a cost of $2.73 each day to hear well. I remind San Franciscans that this is less than the cost of traveling over the Golden Gate Bridge every morning. Similarly a pair of $4,000 hearing aids cost $2.19 per day (less than a Big Mac and fries), and $3,000 worth of hearing aids cost $1.64 per day (about the price of a gallon of supreme gasoline in Northern California). You can devise similar comparisons unique to your geographic locale.

HEARING AID ORIENTATION

The "trial period" discussed earlier might as well be called the "hazard" period unless the patient has (1) received appropriate orientation, and (2) created realistic expectations. New hearing aids provide the ears (and ultimately the brain) with a novel set of stimuli that require an adjustment period. In addition to detailed instruction regarding the proper use and maintenance of new hearing instruments, patients must be counseled about how they should "break-in" their new devices, how they should implement the new set of listening behaviors that should accompany amplification, and what they should and should not expect their new hearing aids to do. Failure to establish realistic expectations may be one of the most prevalent, yet preventable, reasons for returned-for-credit devices. Most hearing aid users have lost their hearing gradually. The status quo for them, or what they consider "normal," is not normal by the normal listener's standards. In fact, the patient's standard of "normal" hearing has changed through the years and is the hearing with which he walked into your office. Therefore, even if the patient demonstrates benefit from amplification, he may still lack satisfaction. Hearing aid patients may forget that they couldn't hear *perfectly* in a restaurant prior to losing their hearing, yet now they think they should. The middle-aged or elderly patient would never expect a new shoe design to allow him to run as fast or jump as high as he could at age 25; yet, he fully expects the hearing aids to restore the hearing he recalls having back then. In Chapter 7, Elaine Mormer and Catherine Palmer propose a detailed orientation program and strategy to establish realistic goals and expectations for hearing aid users.

USE OF SUBJECTIVE AND OBJECTIVE OUTCOME MEASURES AS COUNSELING TOOLS

Evolving managed care guidelines have forced audiologists to validate the effectiveness of their treatments. When insurers agree to pay for a treatment (e.g., hearing aids) they want proof that their subscribers are actually obtaining satisfaction from the provider. Several factors comprise satisfaction. Cox (1997) estimates that satisfaction is comprised of 40% benefit (both psychosocial and acoustic), 25% personal image, 19% service and cost, and 16% negative features. The treatment (hearing aids and/or aural rehabilitation) can be considered successful only if it reduces communication difficulties, enhances psychosocial well-being, and produces functional improvements that remain long after the initiation of rehabilitation (Weinstein, 1996). The use of both objective and subjective outcome measures can be employed to verify whether these objectives have been achieved.

Although outcome measures have generally been designed for validation purposes, they also can be valuable as counseling tools. They can help in assessing whether goals have been met and whether expectations have been realistic. Improper use of outcome measures also can hinder the rehabilitative process. Numerous outcome measures can be applied to hearing aid-related validation. Several of these are mentioned in Chapter 8. It is beyond the scope of this chapter to discuss all of the available gauges. However, because outcome measures have become so pervasive in our practices, and because they represent a significant tool for counseling (one that doesn't fit neatly into any of the other chapters), I will discuss a few of the more commonly used measuring devices here. These measures can be classified as either objective or subjective. Examples of objective measures include the use of prescriptive target formulas, word recognition scores, or functional gain. Subjective measures (many of which can be found in the Appendixes following Chapter 8) include scales such as the Hearing Handicap Inventory for the Elderly (HHIE) (Ventry & Weinstein, 1982) or Hearing Handicap Inventory for Adults (HHIA) (Newman, Weinstein, Jacobson, and Hug, 1991), the Abbreviated Profile of Hearing Aid Benefit (APHAB) (Cox & Alexander, 1995), the Hearing Aid Performance Inventory (HAPI) (Walden, Demorest, & Hepler, 1984; Schum, 1992), the Client Oriented Scale of Improvement (COSI) (Dillon, James, and Ginis, 1997), and the Patient Expectations Worksheet described by Mormer and Palmer in Chapter 7.

Objective Measures as Counseling Tools

Word Recognition Scores

Carhart's classic selection methods (1946) persisted in their popularity for over 30 years, until the advent of probe microphone measures. The concept of selecting the best amplification system for an individual on the basis of a comparison among monosyllabic word recognition scores was generally unchallenged until researchers proved statistically that true superiority of one system over another required differences in word recognition scores that were quite substantial (Thornton & Raffin, 1978), and even then, did not necessarily equate with patient preference. Most dispensers today question the effectiveness of word recognition scores as valid determinants of hearing aid performance, yet patients still occasionally request measurement of word recognition scores as a means of determining if they are "really" doing better with their new hearing aids. When these measures are used, there are several issues that must be considered, particularly with regard to using these data to counsel patients. First, make certain there is room for improvement over unaided scores. A patient scoring over 90% in quiet unaided is not likely to demonstrate improved scores with hearing aids. Furthermore, when little or no improvement is demonstrated, the patient's initial reaction to amplification can be seriously damaged. Therefore, it is essential to degrade the speech signal sufficiently so that the unaided performance will be less than optimal. This can be done with background noise, but the risk is that the same signal-to-noise (S/N) ratio needed to degrade the unaided score will preclude measurable aided benefit. Bentler, Humes, and Cox (1998) have shown that in extremely noisy conditions even the most technologically advanced hearing systems do not demonstrate benefit over crude listening contraptions when measured by word recognition scores.

There are also questions concerning the face validity of monosyllabic words; thus, sentence tests have enjoyed a recent increase in popularity. As a result, many clinicians have opted for measuring the signal-to-noise ratio at which the listener can achieve 50% word recognition. Here, patients can be counseled that even a small improvement (i.e., a 2 dB improvement aided vs. unaided S/N), can translate into as much as a 20% difference in the real world.

Functional Gain

Patients who are familiar with reading audiograms may request confirmation of benefit by viewing evidence of improved sensitivity. Before allowing the patient to view functional gain (the difference between aided and unaided threshold), the limitations of this approach should be discussed. Patients need to be informed, in lay terms, that because these measures are made at threshold, the hearing aids may not be operating with the same compression characteristics that would be functioning during typical listening situations. In other words, gain could be overestimated, because for many hearing aids having low compression kneepoints (e.g., in wide dynamic range compression systems) gain is highest for softer input levels. Conversely, gain can be underestimated because the amount of improvement in aided thresholds may be limited by the ambient noise level, even in a sound-treated booth. This noise floor may be high enough to produce masking, thus elevating the true aided threshold if thresholds are particularly good (i.e., better than 20 dB HL).

Probe Microphone Targets

Probe microphone measures provide an objective and visually engaging measure of the amount of gain and/or output provided by the hearing aid. The audiologist has a choice of several formulas. When the target is "hit," patients are generally quite pleased (even prior to testing out the amplification system in the real world). On the other hand, if you're going to allow the patient to believe that the "correct" amount of gain and frequency response is that which matches the target, you had better be certain you can reach the target. If you know you cannot achieve the target, don't enter the threshold into the analyzer. For example, if the patient presents thresholds of 20 dB at 2000 Hz and 110 dB at 8000 Hz, and the prescriptive formula calls for insertion gain of 6 dB at 2000 Hz and 50 dB at 8000 Hz, it is highly unlikely that the target can be achieved. Therefore, it is advisable to not enter in these thresholds, or select different formulas that are attainable. Also remember to explain to the patient that gain will vary as a function of input level. Given the fact that most digital and programmable hearing aids employ compression (and many no longer contain volume controls), a single input level is not sufficient to define their function. That is why it is wise to employ a few input intensities to simulate soft speech (45 dB SPL), conversational speech (65 dB SPL), and loud speech (85 dB SPL). Explain that the target you are aiming for will vary depending on the input intensity. Also, remember that although observation of the relationships of these curves may verify that the compression is working, it does not verify that the 45 dB SPL input signal is audible, the 65 dB SPL input signal is comfortable, or the 85 dB SPL input is loud, but not uncomfortable. Many of today's prescriptive formulas such as FIG 6 and DSL [i/o], make these assumptions based on average group data, but none of these has been validated. Thus, subjective statements must be elicited from the individual patient to substantiate these conclusions.

Furthermore, the patient needs to be advised that matching a target gain recommended by a prescriptive formula or computer-specified algorithm is only the initial step in the fitting process. Fine-tuning beyond the specified target is essential if the user's acoustic needs are to be met. Remind the patient that personal preferences (i.e., comfort vs. audibility) should override formula data, at least for the initial fitting.

An alternative approach to matching targets uses the DSL [i/o] (Cornelisse, Seewald, & Jamieson, 1995) program to generate the patient's thresholds and uncomfortable loudness levels (UCLs) in SPL. In this way, real ear aided response curves can be plotted against the individual's dynamic range, and the patient can be visually shown this relationship.

Patients need to be advised that benefit from hearing aids is not simply a function of improved word recognition scores or enhanced functional or real ear gain. Each listener has his own unique definition of benefit, and this definition should be established before deciding on the appropriate outcome measure. Once it has been determined, assessment should be conducted using subjective methods.

Subjective Measures as Counseling Tools

Even when targets are matched, audibility is achieved, and word recognition scores are improved, patients may continue to express dissatisfaction with their new hearing instruments. It might be convenient to blame this discontent on unrealistic expectations, but the reality is that even when it appears that the patient, with the guidance of the audiologist, has established realistic expectations, lack of satisfaction may persist. It is important to remember that (1) satisfaction is made up of factors other than benefit, and (2) the concept of "normalcy" that the patient may be striving for may be different from what the audiologist or the normal-hearing person would term normal. Counseling based on the results of subjective outcome measures can help overcome complaints such as "sounds are unnatural."

A variety of psychometrically valid subjective measures can be used as counseling tools. Selection of which measure should be put to use may depend on the point you are trying to prove. For example, if you are trying to illustrate the amount of benefit a patient is receiving, you might use the APHAB, HHIE, or HAPI. Getting even more specific, if you want to measure subjective benefit for speech in quiet, you might employ the Q subscale from the HAPI or the EC (ease of communication) subscale from the APHAB. If you want to measure subjective benefit for speech in noise, you might employ the N subscale from the HAPI or the BN (background noise) or RV (reverberation) subscales from the APHAB. If you wish to assess a reduction in the patient's perceived hearing handicap, the HHIE-S (a 10-item screening test scored on a 1–4 scale per item) is a good choice. Or, as discussed in Chapter 7, to determine whether the patient's goals or expectations were met, you can use the COSI or the Patient Expectation Worksheet, respectively. It also is important that you understand how much of a change in score is needed to represent a true change in the variable being measured. For example, from a statistical perspective, a patient must have a change in score of at least 10 (out of a maximum of 40) on the HHIE-S to be considered a significant reduction in handicap. Or, an APHAB subscale score must improve by 22 points, or the EC, BN, and RV must each improve by 5 points to be considered significant.

Parenthetically, one might question whether a change in subjective re-action has to be statistically significant in order to be meaningful to a patient's perception, or perhaps more important, to contributing to a patient's confidence level during the critical adjustment period.

An effective method of utilizing outcome measures in counseling is to demonstrate to the patient the relative amount of benefit he is receiv-ing compared to the amount of disability reduction received by other individuals facing similar situations (Cox (1997). For example, the APHAB software can generate graphs depicting the percentage of problems experienced by a patient versus those experienced by mem-bers of similar groups. Among the groups available for comparison are (1) linear hearing aid users, (2) elderly patients reporting few or no hearing problems, and (3) young normal-hearing adults. Thus, the au-diologist can demonstrate to a geriatric patient who complains that he is not receiving as much benefit as he thinks he should in noise, that the percentage of time he experiences difficulty hearing in noise is now (with amplification) no different than other elderly patients who report few or no hearing problems. Remember that, as referred to in the dis-cussion of the use of unaided versus aided word recognition scores, you won't see improvements when the patient is already at ceiling level on a scale (i.e., has minimal trouble to begin with). So when using measurement scales, explain to the patient that improvements in the extreme conditions (i.e., in quiet or in excessive noise) are not likely to be seen.

For patients who complain about abnormal loudness, it might be useful to administer the Profile of Aided Loudness (PAL) test (Mueller & Palmer, 1998). This 1–7 loudness scale provides an indication of how the aided listener rates the loudness of soft, average, and loud sounds compared to ratings of the same sounds by normal listeners. It may be, for example, that a patient rates the background hum from a refrigera-tor as a 2 (same as a normal listener) but he may still find it to be annoyingly loud. Then, it should be explained to the patient that be-cause this sound is novel to him (assuming he wasn't hearing it without his hearing aids), his brain isn't suppressing it yet. This is another re-minder that we hear in our brain, not in our ears. It is likely that, in time, the brain will adapt to this unimportant signal so that it is not perceived as much. If, on the other hand, the patient rated that signal as a 4, then indeed it is likely that adjustments would have to be made to the hearing aids. Or, the patient may describe a siren as being very loud (thus disturbing), but because that is the intent of the sound, the patient's judgment would be "just right."

Another use of outcome measures that can be used to improve counseling skills was described by Palmer (personal communication,

1998). She compared the percentage of listening situations in which hearing aid users (1) exceeded their expectations, (2) met their expectations, and (3) fell below their expectations. Using data in this manner can help gauge if you are guiding your patients toward realistic expectations. If you determine that your patients' expectations are consistently not being met, then either you need to counsel for lowered expectations or try different hearing aids or fitting techniques.

LONG-TERM REHABILITATION

Hearing and listening are close cousins of each other, but are not synonymous. Once patients have been given the tools to help them hear, it is the job of the audiologist to help them develop long-lasting expertise to augment their listening abilities. Teaching patients to comprehend the general meaning of spoken messages by using situational and linguistic cues is essential to their long-term use of amplification. Patients should be taught to:

1. listen intently
2. show interest while others are talking (using eye contact and body language)
3. absorb the speaker's mood
4. use closure and guessing skills
5. formulate statements summarizing the speaker's statements
6. accept corrections easily
7. utilize coping strategies to improve redundancy (repeating, rephrasing, confirming, etc.)
8. disregard distractions and noise
9. don't give up prematurely
10. analyze errors in listening strategy

The convergence of hearing aid use, speechreading, assistive listening devices, controlling of auditory environment, and "training" of family members comprise audiologic rehabilitation. The format for teaching these skills can be either individual or group. Many professionals fail to provide this final piece of the rehabilitation puzzle because they fear it will require too much time, preparation, and materials, and will be cost ineffective. In Chapter 8, Kathy Matonak presents an in-depth discussion of long-term rehabilitation. In addition, recognizing the time and cost associated with establishing a curriculum for such programs, Matonak has compiled sample curriculums and an extensive Appendix of materials that can be immediately employed in your own program.

SPECIAL CHALLENGES OF COUNSELING PARENTS OF CHILDREN WHO ARE HEARING IMPAIRED

It is complicated to counsel and reason with certain adult patients in order to get them to take the necessary steps to improve their lives through better hearing. But, at least with adults, we are usually dealing directly with the patients. Undertaking rehabilitative (or habilitative) services with children presents its own special set of counseling challenges because, not only are we forced to work through intermediaries (parents or guardians), but we may also be trying to obtain information from patients who are unable to communicate their feelings to us. Moreover, the effects on emotions and family dynamics present in circumstances surrounding hearing impaired adults are often magnified in those involving hearing impaired children. For example, the difficulty parents may have accepting the fact that their child has a permanent impairment may interfere with logical thinking. Thus, the audiologist must be able to combine empathy and firmness in order to prepare parents to move forward in their child's behalf. The proper use and understanding of adjunctive materials (e.g., reading materials, videotapes, organizations, support groups, financial support, and laws governing the rights of children with disabilities) are essential. Different strategies must be employed in overcoming a child's resistance to wearing hearing aids that might be caused by a multitude of factors, not all of which are related to the child. Thus, in Chapter 9, Becky Bingea considers the unique aspects of counseling parents of children who are hearing impaired. At the end of that chapter, a comprehensive list of support materials, resources, organizations, educational options, and laws governing amplification and education for hearing impaired children is presented.

DEALING WITH THE "CHALLENGING" PATIENT

The final chapter in this book deals with the darker side of audiology and hearing aid fittings that we don't often like to consider when we are trying our best to help hearing impaired patients. But, unfortunately, as with any segment of society, there are those individuals who tax us and push us to our personal and financial limits. They are the patients who challenge our methods and our altruistic wills. In Chapter 10, Joyce Johnson, Lori Pakulski, and Helena Solodar present case histories and review strategies for dealing with these "challenging" patients.

CONCLUSIONS

The modern world we live in has produced increased pressures and decreased time to attend to those things most important to us. When patients put their trust in us they are asking for much more than a pair of electronic devices to place in their ears. They want to know how they can restore the quality of life they once had before they or someone they love had his world altered by a hearing impairment. Hearing aids have become so complicated that even professionals have difficulty keeping up with the rapid changes and ever-increasing options in the field. Patients certainly cannot cut through these tangled webs without professional help. In this introductory chapter, I have outlined the scope of material that will be covered in this book. I hope you will find that the material inspires you to improve your counseling skills, furnishes you with new ideas to enhance your business, and elevates the quality of the services you provide your patients.

REFERENCES

Bentler, R., Humes, L., & Cox, R. (1998). *Hearing Aids. Report form the research front.* Paper presented at a featured session at the American Academy of Audiology meeting, Los Angeles, CA.

Carhart, R. (1946). Tests for the selection of hearing aids. *Laryngoscope,* 56, 780–794.

Cornelisse, L., Seewald, R., & Jamieson, D. (1995). The input/output formula: A theoretical approach to the fitting of personal amplification devices. *Journal of the Acoustical Society of America,* 97(3), 1854–1864.

Cox, R., & Alexander, G. (1995). The Abbreviated Profile of Hearing Aid Benefit. *Ear and Hearing,* 16, 176–186.

Cox, R. (1997). Administration and application of the APHAB. *The Hearing Journal,* 50(4), 32–48.

Cox, R. (1997). *Satisfaction from Amplification for Daily Living (SADL).* Paper presented at the University of California, San Francisco Audiology/Amplification Update III, San Francisco, CA.

Dillon, H., James, A., & Ginis, J. (1997). Client oriented scale of improvement (COSI) and its relationship to several other measures of benefit and satisfaction provided by hearing aids. *Journal of the American Academy of Audiology,* 8, 27–43.

Mueller, G., & Palmer, C. (1998). The Profile of Aided Loudness. A new "PAL" for '98. *Hearing Journal, 51*(1), 10–19.

Newman, C., & Levitt, H. (1990). Selection procedures for digital hearing aids. *Seminars in Hearing, 11*(1), 79–89.

Newman, C., Weinstein, B., Jacobson, G., & Hug, G. (1991). Test-retest reliability of the Hearing Handicap Inventory for Adults. *Ear and Hearing, 12,* 135–137.

Pascoe, D., (1980). Clinical implications of nonverbal methods of hearing aid selection and fitting. *Seminars in Hearing, 1,* 217–229.

Schum, D. (1992). Responses of elderly hearing aid users on the Hearing Performance Inventory. *Journal of the American Academy of Audiology, 3,* 3008–3014.

Thornton, A.R., & Raffin, M.J. (1978). Speech discrimination scores modeled as a binomial variable. *Journal of Speech and Hearing Research, 21,* 507–518.

Ventry, I., & Weinstein, B. (1982). Identification of elderly people with hearing problems. *ASHA, 25,* 377–341.

Walden, B.E., Demorest, M.E., & Hepler, E.L. (1984). Self-report approach to assessing benefit derived from amplification. *Journal of Speech and Hearing Research, 27,* 49–56.

Weinstein, B. (1996). Treatment efficacy: Hearing aids in the management of hearing loss in adults. *Journal of Speech and Hearing Research, 39*(5), S37–S45.

Carole Shelton and Rosemary Faucette are our first guides on this journey into the process of integrating hearing aids with comprehensive hearing rehabilitation. Simply instructing reluctant patients that they must wear hearing devices is a woefully inadequate approach. Resistance to wearing instruments and denial of communication problems are common behaviors among patients who are hearing impaired and must be overcome prior to the initiation of hearing aids into the rehabilitation process. In the ensuing chapter, the authors detail a technique that encourages patients to become active partners in the selection and fitting of hearing aids. The method promoted by Shelton and Faucette entails eliciting both emotional and practical descriptions of the impact that hearing loss exerts on psychosocial aspects of patients' lives in an effort to motivate and prepare them for the upcoming rehabilitative effort. Their approach enlists patients as part of the rehabilitative "team," allowing them to reach conclusions about the importance of hearing in general and the pros and cons of the use of hearing aids.

2

Preparing the Patient for Amplification

■ Carole W. Shelton, M.A. ■
■ Rosemary Faucette ■

Historically, hearing aid companies have poured millions of dollars into the development of higher quality hearing aids. It was assumed that better hearing aids would increase user satisfaction and, thus, increase sales of amplification systems. Has it worked?

Have the number of hearing aid users grown relative to the number who need them? No.

Have hearing aid return rates fallen significantly? No.

Are users as satisfied as hearing professionals hoped they would be? No.

We have to ask ourselves, "Why Not?"

Patients frequently view the decision to wear amplification as a forced one. Nagging spouses, concerned friends, or uncomfortable circumstances have commonly prompted patients to investigate hearing aid use. Once in the office, they find themselves barraged with information, and 1 hour later they exit the office with contract in hand, but doubts in their heads.

Conversely, patients engaging in a deliberate process of full-spectrum thinking, guided by the dispenser, can empower themselves to make the decision not only to purchase the instruments, but to wear them. This deliberate exploration expands the dispenser's role from information-giver (sage on the stage) to facilitator (guide on the side).

Directed Discovery is the term we will use in this chapter to describe a process for thinking about hearing loss and the decision to wear amplification. It entails attitudinal, analytical, and objective thinking. This process is derived from the works of researchers and educators and is based on psychologic and neuropsychologic principles. The brain acts as a self-organizing system. It takes in data and systematically categorizes it into larger patterns or perceptive tracks. This enables humans to make meaning of their environment, and this is good. The downside is that once the brain associates any information with a particular pattern, one may become stuck in that pattern. How does this relate to preparing patients for change? Simply put, most patients walk into the dispenser's office with an already-established perspective on their hearing loss and hearing aid use. What mental image do most people associate with hearing loss? Old age! Right, old people wear hearing aids. What association do people attach to old age? Usually not a very positive one. Thus, many patients walking into your office already have adopted a negative pattern of thinking about their hearing loss and their need for a hearing device. They are likely to maintain this negative pattern unless we, as guides, help them discover alternate ways of thinking.

This can be done, in part, by directing the patient's brain to compartmentalize his thinking, exploring one "compartment" fully before moving on to the next. The brain cannot effectively look at all sides of a picture simultaneously, somewhat like a compass cannot point in all directions at once. In effect, we say to the patient, *"Let's look at your hearing loss from* **this** *direction. When we have fully explored that perspective, we will change direction, again thoroughly exploring* **that** *view."* The dispenser helps the patient repattern his thinking process so that he can clarify his thinking.

Without properly structured guidance, the brain functions like a pinball, bouncing from thought to thought, and, unfortunately, our counseling with the patient may proceed in the same way. In one discussion, the patient may talk about how his hearing loss occurred, how he feels about it, what he thinks he wants to do about it, but why that might not work. Information is thus gathered but in a scattered and disjointed manner. Also, there is information the patient may consciously or subconsciously withhold. At the same time, he may provide information that is of little importance to the final outcome.

By using traditional counseling strategies alone, the patient may never view this conversation as leading to an empowered decision. As counselors, we have focused on identifying the problems, recommending solutions, and seeing that they are implemented. The patient has played a very passive role. He sat; he listened; he followed (or not). With this alternative counseling strategy (guide on the side), the patient is actively involved in thinking through the pertinent issues, and he renders a decision that is solely his. He talks; he processes; he decides.

Furthermore, it is human nature to approach new ideas tentatively. We often regard the negative aspects, why something *won't* work, more powerfully than the positive aspects, why it *will*. Structured guidance can "unstick" this pattern.

A combination of traditional counseling techniques with Directed Discovery can help focus your patient's thinking and change his mind from the perspective he entered with into a multidimensional overview about his hearing loss and the wearing of hearing instruments. This will empower him to move toward an acceptance of his hearing loss, the need for hearing aids, and the ultimate consistent use of these devices.

OVERVIEW OF DIRECTED DISCOVERY

Directed Discovery requires a shift in the dispenser's role from that of lecturer to that of facilitator. The following explanation of this process may seem complex. However, the application of the process is quite short, requiring only minutes in each segment.

Inventory of Feelings: Rationale

Attitudinal Thinking

We start the Directed Discovery process with this premise:

> **Purchasing and wearing hearing aids is an emotional decision. Unless dealt with effectively, emotions will sabotage the entire process.**

People often do not value acknowledging feelings. We engage in a system of polarity, believing some feelings to be "good," and therefore comfortable to be shared, and others to be "bad." These are the ones we keep locked up, refusing to identify, much less honor. So, patients may not readily admit that embarrassment, fear, and insecurity are silent partners that accompany them into the room.

Think of "bad" feelings metaphorically as the whiny child, tugging on his mother's coattails. The more he is ignored, the louder and more insistent he becomes. His power to distract and to sabotage grows. What the child needs, what our "bad" feelings need, is to be honored—to be acknowledged. So, leading the patient through a brief exercise to identify those intrusive, subconscious feelings is the first step. By helping him identify and honor all emotions related to the hearing loss and hearing aids, the dispenser provides a structured "release" for these negative emotions; they are out in the open and can no longer sabotage his conscious efforts. Traditionally, dispensers have not recognized the importance of this emotional component, and thus, the importance of attitudinal thinking to the entire decision-making process.

Next, Directed Discovery focuses the patient on the positive emotions associated with the decision to *wear* amplification: self-respect, hope, courage, satisfaction. When we help him focus on the positive feelings, we lessen the power the negative feelings may have had. Because you have established yourself as caring about the patient's feelings, not just the hearing loss, you immediately establish rapport and the trust that accompanies it. With traditional counseling strategies, we may also have established rapport. We encouraged the patient to trust our expertise in choosing the best solution to correct his hearing problem. Thus, we indeed achieved our short-term goal: that the patient *purchases* hearing devices. By failing to recognize the importance of the emotional component, however, we stop short of fulfilling our responsibility to long-range goals: that the patient leaves our office with a more expanded *understanding* of his situation and a commitment to *purchase* and *to wear* hearing devices on a consistent basis.

If you spend time more effectively dealing with these emotional roadblocks, you will spend less time chasing phantom problems and solutions. By spending your time in this exploratory process, you will create an atmosphere where the patient can

- *explore* all his feelings
- *express* them freely
- *honor* their existence and put them into proper perspective

Inventory of Expectations: Rationale

Analytical Thinking

The next step in Directed Discovery is the "Benjamin Franklin Close," a business term that you may recognize as the traditional pro/con list.

The reason the dispenser directs the patient through this exercise is to help him identify and distinguish between the advantages and disadvantages of wearing hearing devices. Although the patient may have thought through some of the pros and cons, he has likely done it in a haphazard way. Without this structure provided by the dispenser, he never was able to see them listed, side by side, as compartmentalized subjects. Therefore, the conclusions he has drawn may have been unduly weighted by the preexisting negative patterns.

Remember, the patient can easily identify every reason under the sun why wearing hearing amplification will not work for him. We are all quite facile at listing the negatives. Because it is harder to do, it is important to focus *first* on the benefits of hearing devices.

This is where you establish the "thinking team," comprised of the patient, the dispenser, and perhaps a family member who has accompanied the patient. You will act not only as guide but also as scribe, writing down (within the patient's sight) every positive or negative aspect he or his partner identify.

Writing each point gives concrete form to abstract ideas. It also provides validity to and acceptance of the patient's thinking. Again, it says to the patient his ideas are important, that you are there not to sell or to persuade, but to listen. Vital to this process is the idea of focusing *only* on the advantages at one point and disadvantages at another.

Inviting the significant other to contribute increases the synergy and lets the patient know he is not alone in this process. It is important to act only as scribe, resisting the urge to contribute to the list until the patient has exhausted all of his ideas. Affirmations like "Good, Right, Yes," will encourage him to generate as many positive features as possible. Tools to elicit statements will be described shortly.

By engaging the patient and the spouse in this proactive process, you empower the patient. He will ultimately see this as *his* decision, one reached through a structured thinking process.

Delivery of Information: Rationale

Objective Thinking

In this phase of the process, the dispenser presents the necessary information regarding the patient's specific needs and how his expectations should be modified to meet anticipated limitations. Issues such as poor discrimination scores, unusual audiometric configurations, anatomical considerations, and so forth are addressed in this portion of the session. The dispenser affirms the patient's thoughts and conclusions that are consistent with the dispenser's anticipated outcome. She affirms with reservations that thinking that is basically correct but needs further explanation. She corrects misinformation and misperceptions. It is important for the dispenser to present only the information that is in response to the patient's needs or his specific inquiry. In doing so, the patient will more readily recall the data because it has been connected to his thinking.

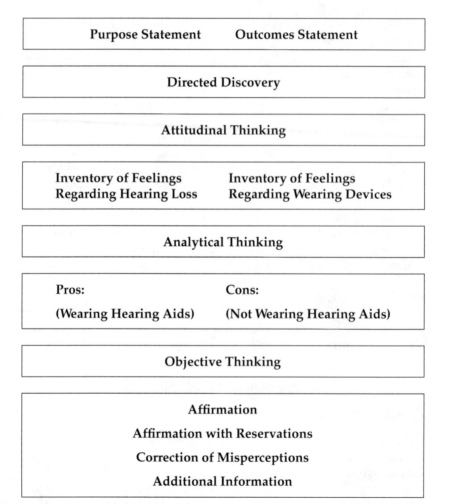

Figure 2–1. Framework of patient/dispenser session

In summary (see Figure 2–1), we use Directed Discovery to

1. Elicit and explore the emotions involved in having a hearing loss and deciding to seek remediation.
2. Form a "thinking team" (we) rather than a confrontational relationship (patient vs. dispenser).
3. Create an inventory of benefits and disadvantages of wearing hearing instruments so that the patient will recognize the worth of proceeding through the process.
4. Provide the dispenser with critical information about the patient.
5. Provide the patient with critical information, correct misinformation about his hearing loss, and develop a realistic idea of what he can expect from hearing instruments.

In this Directed Discovery process, the goal is to help the patient change his perception of his hearing loss in order to create a successful long-term outcome. To do that, dispensers must deal with the emotionally charged issues of hearing loss and expand ways of accessing patient thinking.

ANALYSIS OF THE PATIENT/DISPENSER COUNSELING SESSION

Table 2–1 presents the counseling schedule. The following discussion illuminates the components.

Dispenser Preparation

Dispenser Focusing Exercise

As the dispenser, you must prepare yourself mentally to lead your patient through a focused process. If you are distracted, tired, or cranky, you will be less effective in your ability to guide the patient. Spend a few minutes focusing on your purpose and outcome, letting nothing else interfere. If it helps, make a list of those distractions (sick child at home, car payment due, reports not written, orders not placed, etc.) on a slip of paper and set it aside. Subconscious agendas can influence patient-dispenser rapport negatively.

Environmental Scan

The dispenser should look around the office/examining room space and ask, What is in this space that might affect the patient positively or

Table 2–1. Schedule of the Patient/Dispenser Session

Dispenser Preparation	Time: 5 minutes
Environmental Scan	
Professional Image Check	
Patient Profile Review	
Dispenser Focusing Exercise	
Time Management	
Patient Greeting	Time: 2 minutes
Body Language	
Mirroring Techniques	
The Patient You Don't See	
Introduction	Time: 2 minutes
Purpose and Outcomes Statement	
Body Language	
Directed Discovery Process Begins	
1. First Use of Attitudinal Continuum	Time: 5 minutes
Inventory of Opinions (Feelings)	
First Focus: Hearing Loss	
Second Focus: Hearing Aids	
2. Inventory of Patient's Expectations	Time: 8 minutes
The Benjamin Franklin Close: Pros/Cons	
Comparison of Total Number	
3. Second Use of Attitudinal Continuum	Time: 1 minute
4. Presentation of Information	Time: 5 minutes
Affirmation	
Affirmation with Reservations	
Correction of Misperceptions	
Additional information	
5. Final use of Attitudinal Continuum	Time: 2 minutes
	Total time: 30 minutes

negatively? Is it tidy and organized? Are instruments and papers from previous patients lying around? Are there informational brochures within sight that might interest or distract the patient? How is the seating arranged? When given the choice, some patients will choose a more formal configuration that separates them from the dispenser by a desk. Others may prefer a more casual arrangement whereby the two are seated in closer proximity, with the desk (barrier?) off to the side. If possible, place chairs in both positions and watch where the patient chooses to sit. This bit of "body language" can provide important attitudinal information. Choosing to seat himself in close proximity to the dispenser may indicate his expectations for a more informal manner while a seated position across a desk may indicate a desire for a more professional approach.

Professional Image

The way you dress is, of course, a statement of individuality. In our society, however, most people expect those with whom they do business to dress professionally. Wearing jeans, when the patient expects more formal attire, may send the wrong message to the patient. For this reason, professional dress is the rule rather than the exception. You may even want to keep the old white coat handy. Years of exposure to the medical field have led some patients to expect this degree of formality, even among allied professions. On the other hand, the white coat approach may scare certain patients (particularly young children who may have had unpleasant experiences, such as injections, at the doctor's office). If you fail to recognize the potential attitudinal variations in your patient base, you may be making more of a statement than you intended.

Patient Profile Review

Some patients will, of course, be completely new to you. Note any information previously obtained: audiograms, questionnaires, rescheduled or canceled appointments, and prior contacts with your office. This information will allow you to prepare for specific limitations (poor word recognition abilities, problematic audiometric configurations, etc.) that you will need to address as you guide him toward choosing the most appropriate hearing instruments. Canceled or rescheduled appointments may indicate a reluctance to pursue remediation.

Also, mentioning to your patient some seemingly trivial item of information will convey to him that you have familiarized yourself with his specifics, seeing him as an individual rather than merely the next name in your appointment calendar.

Dispenser: I see by your file that you saw Sylvia last time you were in our office or, I see that you had to cancel your last two appointments. I'm glad we finally were able to get our schedules together.

Time Management.   When you arrive late for a scheduled appointment, it says to the patient, "My time is more important than yours." We expect the patient to arrive promptly, and yet we are often tempted to make one more phone call, finish up a report, or complete an unfinished order. Although patients sometimes recognize the inevitable delays in medical offices, you should make every effort to manage your time so that no patient has to wait more than 5 minutes. Promptness implies that you respect his time and that you are efficient and organized in your business dealings.

Patient Contact

It is of critical importance to establish a good working rapport with the patient from the first point of contact. We must quickly establish ourselves as having the knowledge, the desire, and the ability to help the patient effect the changes required to improve communication. The patient must *trust* us—*trust* that we will use the information he imparts in a nonjudgmental way and *trust* that we care about the eventual outcome. Evaluation of body language and mirroring techniques are tools dispensers use to develop this rapport.

Body Language

Reading body language is a two-way street. When you greet the patient, be aware of the messages you are projecting with your own unconscious body language. The patient's impression of you should be one of quiet confidence. Be aware of your **gestures.** Confident individuals usually keep their hands still or make gestures with their hands and body that are meaningful and deliberate. Good **eye contact** is critical in establishing rapport. It also establishes good modeling, as we encourage the patient to use eye contact to augment his communication. A credible advisor conveys an expression of interest and sincerity when consistently looking into the patient's eyes. Your **voice** should be pitched comfortably low and resonate from the chest. Speaking speed, too, is important. Aim at a rhythm that is fractionally slower than normal. It should not be too fast (which can imply urgency, nervousness, or impatience) or too slow (which can indicate indecisiveness). Most of us experienced in working with people who are hearing impaired are accustomed to speaking slower and slightly louder in order to be understood.

We would recommend to all new audiologists (and some of us old-timers as well) to videotape themselves in counseling sessions as a way of assessing their own body language. Review the tape alone and then with co-workers, requesting comments regarding both the content and presentation of your message.

We should, likewise, be conscious of the messages our patients are sending us! Observing the actions of people can bring you a lot closer to the truth than merely listening to what they say (which might be a cover-up). It is an ongoing process and can be very revealing. As a counselor, you should always be sensitive to the way the patient is reacting to you and the information you're dispersing. From his subconscious behaviors, you can also discern whether he is being candid or protective, helpful or resistant.

Try not to move away or flinch when patients draw near or when they touch you. Conversely, try to judge space accurately so as not to invade the patient's comfort zone. For example, if you lean forward and the patient moves back or tenses up, back off! If you lean back and the individual leans forward, this can indicate an openness and willingness to hear what you have to say. Although it is critical to use physical touch discreetly, it is sometimes helpful to do a "trial touch," that is, a light touch on the arm to gauge the reaction. It's often immediate and gives you great insight to the mind-set of the patient. Some reactions are obvious—a glance at his partner, a furrowing of the brow, or perhaps a smile. Some are not so obvious. The good counselor learns to read those subtle reactions quickly and alters her behavior or presentation to be more acceptable to the patient.

The following list summarizes some subconscious postures you might notice in patient behavior. Although these are generalized conclusions, they should give you the idea that people unwittingly project the inner workings of the mind with outward manifestations.

Openness: Open hands, unbuttoning coat.

Defensiveness: Arms crossed, sideways glance, touching or rubbing nose, rubbing eyes, buttoning coat, pulling away.

Insecurity: Pinching flesh, chewing pen, thumb over thumb, biting fingernails, chewing lip, poor eye contact.

Cooperation: Upper body in sprinter's position, open hands, sitting on edge of chair, hand to face gestures, unbuttoning coat.

Confidence: Steepled hands, hands behind back, back stiffened, hands in coat pockets with thumb out, hands on lapels of coat.

Nervousness: Clearing throat, "whew" sound, whistling, pinching flesh, fidgeting, covering mouth, juggling money or keys, tugging at ears, wringing hands.

Fear: No eye contact—averting eyes to either side of your face, eyes held downward, hand held to brow.

We all have a personality comfort zone in which we operate. This defines who we are. We are not suggesting that all dispensers act alike or assume personalities that are not theirs. However, we should be aware of the subconscious messages we convey with our posture, our eyes, our hands, and our voices.

Mirroring Techniques

A tool for establishing rapport is the use of mirroring techniques. In effect, the patient's behavior—the way he presents himself —"tells" you how you should present yourself to achieve your greatest credibility. If the patient is cool and aloof, assume a similar demeanor, never unfriendly, just matter-of-fact with an emphasis on professionalism. A smile and friendly banter from the patient tells you to project a more casual, lighter attitude. In our office, the patient being evaluated checks in with the receptionist and is seated in the waiting room to be "collected" by the audiologist for the appointment. The greeting and walk back to the hearing aid selection room is about 2 minutes long. The time spent during that short walk can be some of the most productive 2 minutes spent in the entire appointment if used correctly. By the time you reach the designated room, you should have a good idea of how you need to project yourself in order to establish the greatest credibility in the least amount of time. By being sensitive to the patient's projected attitude and mirroring it, within our own comfort range of reactions, we create an environment that fosters trust and assurance.

Name Issues: Mr. or Bob

A general rule of thumb is to address the patient as Mr. (Mrs., Dr., etc.) unless and until instructed by him to do otherwise. Some people find the use of their given name overly familiar and even offensive, especially when addressed by someone significantly younger. One tactic is to introduce yourself by both names and wait to see how he addresses you:

Dispenser: Hello, Mr. Jones. My name is Carole Shelton.

Patient: Hi, Carole. I'm Bob, and this is my wife, Shirley.

The patient has clearly stated that he prefers the use of first names.

If the patient fails to correct this more formal address, however, the dispenser should continue the use of the family name:

Dispenser: Hello, Mr. Jones. My name is Carole Shelton.

Patient: How do you do? I'd like you to meet my wife.

Dispenser: How nice to meet you, Mrs. Jones. I'm so glad you could join us today.

One final note regarding the use of names, particularly when there is a significant age difference between a younger dispenser and older patient. There are some individuals who regard the use of the more formal address as patronizing. Rather than a sign of respect, they see it as being treated as a doddering elder. If you are invited to use the given name, do so, even if you are more comfortable being somewhat deferential. Be aware of the body language and mirror the demeanor of the patient. A lapse in this seemingly small area can damage the easy rapport one strives to establish.

Application of Traditional Techniques

What follows is a model for the initial patient contact.

As you approach your patient, look to see how he is sitting. Is he leaning forward, waiting for your arrival? Or is he relaxed and engrossed in a magazine? Are family members present? Note their postures as well. Are the two relating to each other, or are they seated apart? What information can you infer about this relationship from your observation of their demeanor? Stand about 6 feet away from the patient when you call his name. When he stands, does he approach or does he wait for you to proceed? Who approaches first, the patient or the spouse/partner? How are introductions made? As you proceed toward the examination room, notice if he is beside you or trailing behind. Where is his partner?

You are looking for implied information regarding the degree with which you will engage the spouse in the decision-making process. On whom do you focus first, the patient or the family member?

What is the patient's attitude? Is he jovial and casual, or more formal and aloof? Mirror the demeanor of the patient in your own posture.

Another question you should ask yourself is, "Is there anything about this patient, who appears to be comfortable and determined, that I am not seeing?" It is human nature to present ourselves in the most positive light, and our patients may do just that. Although this is not necessarily a deception, it doesn't always reflect the true nature of patients you are likely to encounter. In other words, don't assume that the person is who he says he is, or believe that he will be forth-right in relating his emotional experience about the hearing loss. You may never know for certain, but you should always be aware of subtle agendas and never assume the story being presented is the complete one.

As you enter the examination room, take your place. Where does the patient sit (provided that there is an option), and where does the partner sit?

You are now ready to get down to business, starting with the introduction of the session, its purpose, and expected outcome. This creates a concrete structure for the patient.

■ The session
   1. Introduction
   2. Statement of purpose
   3. Statement of expected outcomes

Start the formal part of the session by stating a purpose (why you are here) and the desired outcome (what you will have at the end of the session that you do not have now). This is a simple yet powerful act. It focuses both you and the patient. It gives direction. It allows the patient to know exactly *why* he is in your office and *what* he should expect to gain from the session.

The goal of a hearing aid counseling session is twofold:

1. to decide whether the patient wishes to try hearing aids
2. to decide which of the available instruments is most appropriate for him

You may wish to have this purpose statement posted in your office. It is reassuring to the patient to have this structure. He knows where he is going and why. Structures like these, as simple as they may be, provide boundaries of safety. The patient does not have to guess what he is supposed to be doing or saying. He knows all activity has some meaningful direction. He has a way to measure progress. When the decision has been made either way, he knows he has completed the session.

Preparing the patient for Directed Discovery is important as well.

Dispenser: Mr. Smith, by the end of this session we will have made some decisions regarding the choice of hearing devices. I will spend the first few minutes just listening to your opinions and thoughts. So are you ready to begin?

As you proceed into the next segments of the session, the patient will

1. explore his emotional status regarding his hearing handicap
2. assess the pros and cons of wearing amplification
3. receive information that will correct any misperceptions

The result of this is that he will be empowered, feeling less of a victim to the experience.

Armed with information and engaged in the process, the patient will begin to regard himself as an informed partner in the decision. The hearing loss is not so formidable an enemy.

The First Use of Attitudinal Continuum

The purpose of the continuum is to show the patient that his feelings do not have to be totally positive or totally negative and that wherever he places himself on the spectrum, his position is legitimate and acceptable. Offering a range of feelings between the two extremes helps him pinpoint his current status.

We will use this gauge twice more to measure his progress as he broadens his understanding of his hearing loss and its solutions. Keep in mind that opinions change with perception. Directed Discovery will expand his perception base, and, therefore, his initial feelings may change. The following continuum provides this concrete measurement.

Enthusiastic Like Interested Uncertain Misgivings Dislike Hate

The dispenser says,

Mr. Jones, I want you to put an X along this line that best describes your feelings about your **hearing loss.** I'm only going to give you a few seconds so that you don't think about this because there is absolutely no need to justify your feelings. (If appropriate, add) Mrs. Jones, I'd like you to do the same thing on a separate piece of paper. Don't share your papers at this point.

Good, now let's do it again, only this time, I'd like you to circle those words you associate with getting **hearing instruments.**

Put the papers aside with a simple promise to come back to these later. This visual aid will be presented twice more in the session.

The Second Part of Attitudinal Thinking: Eliciting the Patient's Feelings (Opinions) Regarding His Hearing Loss

We have included the option of using the word "opinions" in the place of "feelings." Some people are uncomfortable using the latter. They may find the use of the word "feelings" is unsettling, especially when expressing them to a stranger. You will have received enough feedback from your initial contact with this patient that you can judge the most appropriate approach.

The dispenser says,

Okay, Mr. Jones, I want you to do something else for me. Here is a list of words, some having positive connotations, some having negative connotations. I want you to take 60 seconds and circle the five words that you associate with your **hearing loss.**

Often, a patient does not have a vocabulary for feelings. By presenting him with an "emotional vocabulary" and little time to justify or judge their impact, you will elicit a more candid profile than if you asked him to provide the words himself. Emotions, feelings, and opinions are often invisible roadblocks. Giving them names gets them out in the open where they can be acknowledged. A sample list is presented in Table 2–2.

Stay true to your time frame. Announce that he has 30 seconds left. The brain will do what it is told. He will circle five words in 1 minute. Do not allow more than this amount of time. If you do, it will allow the patient to rationalize his feelings. Again, feelings do not need to be justified. Finding reasons for his thinking will come in the next part of this session.

Now refocus the topic.

Dispenser: Mr. Jones, I want you to do the same thing, but this time circle words that you associate with wearing **hearing aids.**

The purpose of this next exercise is to transform abstract feelings into concrete form.

Dispenser: Give me an example when you have felt that way, or might feel that way.

Do not ask *why* he feels a certain way, as this will require justification. Instead ask *when*. This prompts the patient to tell his story and gives it value.

Sometimes a linguistic framework helps to get him started. Offer this:

Dispenser: When such and such happens, I feel embarrassed . . .

This exercise makes feelings manageable. Identifying feelings by name and pinpointing examples act as release valves. As dispensers, we are not trying to make patients feel better or eradicate the feelings. We are not psychotherapists; we are merely facilitators for the release valves.

Table 2–2. List of Potential Emotional Labels

abandoned	enraged	overwhelmed
accepted	enthused	panicky
aimless	excited	peaceful
alienated	exhausted	powerful
angry	explosive	pressured
annoyed	fearful	proud
anxious	fired up	rebellious
assured	focused	relaxed
betrayed	frightened	remorseful
bewildered	frustrated	responsible
bitter	generous	safe
carefree	gentle	satisfied
cheated	gratified	secure
comfortable	guilty	serene
competent	hassled	sorry
confident	hopeful	spiteful
confused	hopeless	strengthened
content	hostile	strong
curious	impatient	surprised
dedicated	indignant	sympathetic
defensive	inquisitive	tense
delighted	insecure	thoughtful
depressed	inspired	tolerant
disappointed	interested	understood
disciplined	irritated	unloved
discouraged	jittery	unsafe
disgusted	lonely	unsure
dismal	lost	unwanted
disturbed	loved	useless
drained	misunderstood	weary
elated	motivated	wild
empowered	nervous	withdrawn
energetic	obligated	worried

Note: When identifying your feelings, you need not give reasons. Feelings are caused by perception, not logic. Feelings may change as additional thinking creates change in perception.

When you identify your feelings, you should honor them. This acceptance of "what is right now" mollifies the feelings, thus eliminating its insistence to get your attention.

Remember that we are keeping the patient focused *only* on his feelings. The more he can verbalize his feelings, the more they are validated. Assure him that all feelings are legitimate and appropriate.

The dispenser should *never* negate the patient's response.

Dispenser: Oh, you shouldn't feel that way.

It is important at this stage to affirm their legitimacy. Instead, respond with affirming statements.

Dispenser: You're not alone; many people feel this way; yes, I hear this from many people.

A brief dialogue will help the patient express the feeling more fully.

Dispenser: Mr. Jones, let's talk about this word: "Fear." Under what circumstances do you experience fear?

Patient: When I think about getting old.

Dispenser: I see. Anything else?

Patient: No.

Dispenser: Okay, let's move to this next word.

There is no need to have lengthy discussions about each word. Some patients will love the opportunity to share their experiences. For others, a short example is sufficient. If examples become drawn out, an *"I see"* or *"Let's move on to this next word"* is enough of a prompt.

When all the identified words have been amplified, the dispenser may even suggest some the patient failed to circle, especially if you believe that he is holding back or trying to be too accommodating.

Dispenser: You know, a lot of people who do this exercise circle the word, "Anger." Can you cite an example of when you have felt this way, too?

If he says *"No,"* drop it. If he begins to admit to feelings of anger, however, you have "given him permission" to express that feeling and thereby validated it. You have also lightened his burden. You have just told him others report having this feeling as well.

It is important to keep the discussion focused on the patient's feelings, not on the reasons he wants or doesn't want hearing devices. If he starts rationalizing or justifying his feelings, say,

> We will address those issues and more later. Right now we're just talking about how you feel about your hearing loss.

It is important to affirm the patient's "right" to have these feelings, even when they are based on incorrect information or misperceptions.

This entire process should take no longer than 10 minutes. As you become more facile in the Directed Discovery process, the easier it will become. Role-playing with colleagues is excellent practice and will give you confidence and timing.

The Benjamin Franklin Close: Pros and Cons

The purpose of this next step is to engage the patient in listing all the advantages and disadvantages of wearing hearing instruments. Recall that your role is that of facilitator and scribe. As facilitator, you aim the patient's thinking in a singular direction. As scribe, you record the patient's thoughts. This gives them validity. You may give the patient copies of his thinking records to take home for review and to share with family members. This proactive process engages him, empowering him to make that final decision which he alone owns.

Focus the patient's thinking on the advantages first. Listing the positives (the pros) is the more difficult of the exercises, so begin with listing the pros (i.e., If you have two frogs to swallow, swallow the larger one first). By starting with a list of pros, we emphasize the position that wearing hearing devices *will work*. Keep in mind that the patient will naturally want to play the "devil's advocate," so it is important to keep the patient from "veering off" into thinking about both at the same time (i.e., focus, focus, focus). For example, when you are generating ideas in the "pros" column, do not allow "yes-buts" statements such as, *"**Yes,** I think I will hear better, **but** I have to remember to put it on every day."* Listen for the cautionary words "but" and "however" and remind the patient, *"We'll get to the disadvantages later. For now, just list the advantages: 'I think I'll hear better.'"*

Advantages/Pro List

On a piece of paper within the patient's view, number from 1 to 5. This sets an expectation. If you reach 5 easily, add 6 and 7. Keep adding if the patient gets on a roll. But what if the patient stops at 3? Let's emphasize the power of "waiting." Counting to 10 slowly will help you through the dead space, but the silence will shift the responsibility to the patient to continue thinking of merits.

Encourage the patient to give you a specific list of reasons for wearing hearing aids. Trust the process. As dispensers, you already know that the advantages outweigh the disadvantages, but it is important to empower the patient to discover this on his own. Remember, you are not the sage on the stage, only the guide on the side.

Start by saying to the patient:

> We know that being able to hear better is a feature of wearing hearing aids. I would like you to list all the **advantages or merits of hearing better because these are the advantages of hearing aids.**

Don't be concerned if some of his statements seem unrealistic. You will be clarifying misperceptions in the information phase of the session.

The dispenser writes an *abbreviated* form of each response.

For example, he might say:

> I won't have to guess what people are saying. Therefore, I won't appear stupid.
>
> My wife won't complain about the volume of the television, and we can enjoy it together again.
>
> I will be able to participate in discussions, so I won't feel isolated.

Notice there is a cause-and-effect relationship in each statement. The patient will easily be able to give you the *cause*. As the facilitator, **you**

must elicit the *effect* because this is where the advantage lies. It is important for the patient to identify the advantage. If not, he is only listing circumstances.

If the patient seems to be having difficulty, offer a linguistic framework.

> If I hear my wife better, then . . .
> If I hear the television better, then . . .
> If I hear my grandchildren better, then . . .

Again the "if . . . then" linguistic structure sets up the relationship to assist his thinking.

Another way to help generate this list of advantages is to change his point of view. The dispenser asks:

> If your spouse were to record the values of your wearing hearing aids, what things would she list? What about your co-workers?

However, be prepared to suggest advantages not noted by the patient, but always request permission to place them on "his list." For example:

> **Dispenser:** There are a couple of things you didn't put on your list that many people do. Would you mind if I name a few, and if they apply to you, we'll add them. For instance, many people say they will be able to hear their minister better during church services so church will become meaningful once again . Is this something you would include on your list? No? Okay, how about this one? Many folks say hearing clearly at family gatherings is an advantage because now they can participate, no longer feeling like an outsider. Yes? Good. Add that to your list?

Your added suggestions do two things:

1. They expand the list more fully. Patients might forget items of lesser importance, but they become monumental when the hearing aids fail to remedy those situations at home.

2. It will allow you to add situations that, because of the patient's audiologic profile, you know you will have to address later. For example, consider the patient who places "I will hear better at family gatherings" on his list. This patient is known to have both peripheral discrimination and central auditory processing difficulties. You expect the hearing aids will be of limited value in a room full of noisy, chattering relatives. In the **information** portion of this session (not now!) you will address these limitations so that his expectations of clarity (in that situation) are reduced. By including this advantage, you are setting the stage to give him this necessary information later.

Because we are focusing only on positives and not allowing diversions and bird walking (birds don't walk in straight lines), this process requires only about 5 minutes. The dispenser should conclude by listing the number of positive features the "team" has listed. This reinforces to the patient that he has a healthy list of advantages, which affirms his thinking.

Besides bolstering the patient's resolve, this list of advantages will help the dispenser in follow-up appointments. The patient is telling you exactly **why** it is important for him to hear. These are the values he places on hearing aids. So, it is these values that you will continue to reinforce. This framework gives you a personalized benefit assessment profile.

Disadvantages/Con List

Now you are ready to begin the "con" list, asking the patient to point out the reason why wearing a hearing device is not feasible, workable, or beneficial. Again, write down each point the patient makes. Close the "con" list in the same manner, noting the number of negative responses.

At this point you compare the two lists, allowing the patient to see them side by side. Here's where you will have to trust the process. The benefits will outnumber the negatives, a fact the patient may never recognize until he has been guided through a directed assessment. Some people will exclaim with delight, *"Hey, I have 12 positives and only 5 negatives"* With others, it will be necessary to draw attention to the fact that there are more positive features than negatives.

Keep in mind that identifying a disadvantage does not entail reversing an advantage. This may be something you need to tell the patient. When we examine the advantages of wearing hearing aids, we are looking for specific benefits to better hearing. When we examine for disadvantages, we are not seeking the downside of doing nothing. We are identifying the negative aspects of wearing amplification itself.

The framework for generating a list of disadvantages is the same as for the advantages list. Start by numbering from 1 to 5, but be prepared to add on.

The dispenser says:

Okay, Mr. Jones, now, we're going to list on paper all the disadvantages you can identify about wearing hearing aids.

Often, patients will confuse the *effect* of the problem with the *problem.* For instance, a patient responds with, "One of the problems I see is that it will show." He has identified the effect. The real problem lies in the fact that the cosmetic appearance calls unwanted attention and perceived judgment to him. To elicit this disadvantage, respond with, "OK, how is that a problem?" This will usually elicit the disadvantage. For example, he may say, "I will look old or stupid."

Other responses might include:

Patient: Because it might whistle.

Dispenser: OK. Why is this a problem?

Patient: The whistle will draw attention to the hearing device and to me.

Patient: Because it might be uncomfortable

Dispenser: OK. Why is this a problem?

Patient: It might hurt and I won't wear it.

Patient: Because it is expensive.

Dispenser: OK. What is the problem?

Patient: I'd rather spend my money on something else.

Even when the response is based on incorrect information, the dispenser should note it, but should not comment. Correcting misinformation will come later. It is more important to keep the patient engaged in and focused on the thinking.

After a certain number of responses, change the point of view. What problems might your partner or coworker identify?

After that, as you did with the Pro List, offer suggestions that might not have occurred to the patient.

Dispenser: You know, some people think that _____ might present some difficulty. Would that be one you would add to your list?

If he says "yes," again ask him how this would be a problem to him?

The dispenser's overall goal is to create a profile that is patient-specific. Even with prompts, the disadvantages he generates are his own. This aspect of Directed Discovery is what helps the patient make a decision. He has a vested interest in the outcome. He has taken a proactive role in this decision. He is not merely a passive recipient of the dispenser's expertise and knowledge.

To conclude this exercise, we review the lists and point out the *number* of advantages compared to the disadvantages identified by the patient. In the extremely unlikely situation that the cons outnumber the pros, perhaps amplification should be deferred to a later date.

Second Use of the Attitudinal Continuum

At this point we recommend using the continuum as a way to register how the patient is feeling. Because opinions (feelings) change with perception, and because the patient's perception has been expanded through Directed Discovery, his opinions may have been modified. It is important the patient note any attitudinal change.

Enthusiastic Like Interested Uncertain Misgivings Dislike Hate

Presentation of Information

The purpose of this portion of the session is to affirm those patient responses that were based on accurate information, to affirm with reservation and explanation, to identify and correct any misconceptions, and to answer questions the patient may pose.

Affirmation

First, from the pro/con list, select those perceptions that are based on accurate information and are reasonable outcomes.

> **Dispenser:** Looking over these lists, I can see that most of the responses you gave were based on accurate information, and you can indeed expect these outcomes. Better hearing with television, better communication with spouse and friends, more comfort in discussion, less stress, etc. Good for you.

Because the patient will be taking home copies of these exercises, we use a symbol to denote level of accuracy of expectations for the patient to review or reflect.

Use a plus sign (+) beside each of the points that were based on accurate information and are reasonable outcomes. No discussion is needed.

Affirmation with Reservation

Second, select statements that are partially correct, but have limitations to the expected outcome.

> **Dispenser:** Another item you listed was, "I think I will hear better at parties, and if I do, I'll enjoy going to them again instead of staying at home." I have to tell you, though, that understanding speech in a lot of background noise is one the most difficult things to achieve when wearing amplification. I think you will be a lot more comfortable in social situations, but we may have to work on that one. It will be more of a trial-and-error thing, based on the experiences you have once you wear the aids awhile. I'll be able to adjust them (reprogram, etc.), and we'll

also discuss strategies you can use to maximize the listening environment.

Put a check mark (√) next to these items.

Correction of Misperceptions

It is this point in the process where your knowledge, your expertise, your skill as a dispenser may be challenged. This is where you make your mark. This is where you move from facilitator (guide on the side) to teacher (sage on the stage).

Dispenser: However, I noted in a few of your responses, that you formed conclusions that were based on misconceptions or incomplete information. Let me clarify those.

Correction of Item From "Advantage" List

Dispenser: Mr. Jones, you said you expected to hear your pastor's sermon from your position in the choir loft, high in the back of the church. If hearing aids were able to do that, I would be the happiest dispenser in the world. The fact is that the microphone for the hearing aid is in the same position as your ear. The aids are bound to pick up those sounds closest to you more efficiently than those 100 feet away. If Mrs. Jones leafs through her hymnal during the pastor's prayer, you'll likely not hear the prayer. With hearing aids alone, that will continue to be a problem. However, there are assistive listening devices that can help do just exactly what you have described. Let's discuss those options once we have finished selecting your hearing aids.

Notice that in correcting a misperception, the dispenser offers an alternative solution.

Correction of Item from "Disadvantage" List

Dispenser: You mentioned as a disadvantage that the hearing aids might be uncomfortable so you might not wear them. Based on the information you have, I can see how you reached this conclusion. However, these hearing aids are custom fit to your ears. An uncomfortable hearing aid is not acceptable to you or to me. I will work with you to make sure they fit properly. They shouldn't hurt.

Again, contained within the information is the solution. By correcting the perception with accurate information, you may have succeeded in eliminating the problem. Being candid and clear about what he can and cannot expect is vital.

Use as many of the patient's pros/cons as you can as avenues for necessary information. For example, if in one statement he suggests a need for a small apparatus, and in another statement he mentions a need for very powerful hearing aids, his misperception is that he can have both. This may not be true, and you need to give him that information.

Dispenser: You said you wanted hearing aids as small as possible, but you want powerful devices. Sometimes we must choose larger instruments in order to get acceptable power. Which of these is more important to you? Are you able to accept this trade-off?

Again, this information provides empowerment that there may be a trade-off; but it is *his* decision to make, not one you forced on him. The patient now knows there may be a trade-off between power and size, and that he must prioritize his requirements.

We often over-explain solutions by offering scientific theories and concepts that patients simply do not need to know (see Chapter 4). In fact, they often muddle thinking. **Keep it simple, focus on the patient.** Answer only the questions he asks.

For example, patients may ask if they will be able to hear multiple talkers at cocktail parties. For some patients it is unnecessary to explain the importance of high-frequency sounds in the speech spectrum and the overall comprehension of conversation. Tell them the truth.

Dispenser: Probably not as clearly as you want to. Technology just is not there yet.

Finally, invite the patient to ask any questions or present any concerns that may have not yet been addressed. Don't be surprised when the patient has few of either. The Directed Discovery process will have already addressed most of his concerns.

Final Use of Attitudinal Continuum

To achieve closure to the Directed Discovery process, the dispenser directs the patient to reflect on his feelings/opinions again. The process has provided him with many perspectives and necessary information. But it is important that *he* see that his initial feelings/opinions have been modified. To do this, we present the attitudinal continuum one last time. *"So where do you fall on this line now?"* Have him respond (put an X on the line). Many times the patient will note the movement himself. If he does not, the dispenser points it out.

This will mark the transition to the second portion of the appointment (refer to Framework of Session). Note that this entire portion of the session, including the Directed Discovery process, should be completed in no more than 30 minutes.

Dispenser: Are you ready to move on? Shall we take a look at specific devices that will be appropriate for you?

At this juncture, the dispenser's role changes from counselor to technical advisor, presenting and explaining available devices (see Chapters 4 and 5).

SUMMARY

Traditional counseling techniques are important to the establishment of a good rapport between patient and dispenser. A good counselor should be knowledgeable of and skilled in using such techniques as mirroring and reading body language. In this chapter, we have introduced a new concept often unrecognized in the hearing aid dispenser's counseling process: the importance of identifying and honoring the patient's feelings regarding his hearing loss and the use of hearing instruments. By encouraging the patient to explore all his feelings, express them freely, and honor their existence, we help him put those feelings into proper perspective and diffuse their ability to sabotage his conscious thinking processes.

We have also offered a new addition to the dispenser's arsenal, Directed Discovery. This technique directs the patient to think about all the issues involved in the decision to purchase and wear amplification devices in a focused and deliberate manner. By compartmentalizing each of the issues and examining each fully, we allow the patient to prioritize his concerns and address each issue in an organized fashion. This process makes the information he obtains more concrete. It also involves him more fully in the process, making him a critical part of the "thinking team." In this way, he plays a greater role in, and responsibility for, the outcome.

The concepts that distinguish this new paradigm are:

The weight of the responsibility for decisions shifts from the dispenser to the patient.

The focus changes from dispenser-driven discussion to patient-centered exploration.

The dispenser moves from one who controlled the outcome to one who facilitates it.

It will take time to become comfortable and facile in this new mode. Giving information is easy and familiar to most dispensers. There will always be the urge to return to the old ways of counseling. However, we know that they have limitations. We must consider alternate approaches if we truly intend to fulfill our responsibility and meet our desired outcome: **a patient who leaves our office with a more expanded understanding of his situation and a commitment to purchase and to wear hearing devices on a consistent basis.** We also acknowledge that despite the fact that we believe this approach is most appropriate for the majority of patients, we recognize that certain patients do not require the structure or detail of this approach. Experience is the best teacher in determining which patients can forego Directed Discovery.

The idiosyncracies of human behavior are complex. Compounding them with the effect of a sensory impairment to a major sense complicates the matter even further. As Shelton and Faucette indicated in Chapter 2, extracting information from patients so that they can enter the rehabilitative process with a positive perception of the role of hearing aids is essential. In the next chapter, Robert Traynor further highlights the importance of listening to patients and "reading" aspects of their personalities in order to refine counseling efforts. He focuses his discussion on the use of a popular personality inventory tool that has received extensive use in other disciplines and offers a means by which this tool can be employed by hearing health care professionals. It is important to note that even though the particular technique he describes is perhaps too lengthy for regular deployment in a clinical practice, the underlying aspects of the method can improve hearing health care professionals' knowledge of how to approach patients. It also should be recognized that many of the statements made in Chapter 3 regarding classification of individuals are based on supposition rather than validated data from hearing impaired patients. Furthermore, because individual personalities are so complex, there can be dangers in grouping individuals dogmatically, especially on the basis of first impressions. Even so, the information you are about to read should provide you with numerous useful suggestions to help you maximize your efficiency in reaching your patients.

3

Relating to Patients

■ Robert M. Traynor, Ed.D. ■

If I do not want what you want, please do not try to tell me that my want is wrong.

Or if I believe other than you, at least pause before you correct my view.

Or if my emotion is less than yours, or more, given the same circumstances, try not to ask me to feel more strongly or weakly.

Or yet if I act, or fail to act, in the manner of your design for action, let me be.

I do not, for the moment at least, ask you to understand me. That will come only when you are willing to give up changing me into a copy of you.

I may be your spouse, your parent, your friend, or your colleague. If you will allow me any of my own wants, or emotions, or beliefs, or actions, then you open yourself, so that some day these ways of mine might not seem so wrong, and might finally appear to you as right—for me.

To put up with me is the first step to understanding me. Not that you embrace my ways as right for you, but that you are no longer irritated or disappointed with me for my seeming waywardness.

And in understanding me you might come to prize my differences from you, and, from seeking to change me, preserve and even nurture those differences.

Keirsey and Bates (1984)

BASIC ORIENTATION TO PERSONALITY

Audiologists have realized for many years that two patients with the same degree, type, and configuration of hearing impairment do not have the same reactions to their hearing loss. This is evident in that procedures, hearing instruments, earmolds, and other products that provide great benefit for one patient may not be at all beneficial for another. Simultaneously, relating and interacting clinically with the first patient could be quite different from the second. Even though audiologists have been aware of this paradox for the past 40 years, we have conducted rehabilitative treatment with our patients as though they all react to the world exactly the same, but just have a hearing loss. In general, we assume that the hearing loss is causing all the difficulty in relating to the environment without questioning patients' personal styles in their reactions to their world. Because personality style can be quite heterogeneous among humans, it is only reasonable that there can be quite a lot of variability among those who are hearing impaired.

It is not enough to be a good audiologist and a caring available professional. The responsible clinician must attain and maintain the patient's attention for the hearing rehabilitative process to be successful. Methods used by successful audiologists often key on dealing either formally or informally with the patient's personality. As suggested in the introductory quotation, all patients are unique, possessing a special set of formulas by which they interact with the world. If audiologists identify and utilize these unique patient differences, then they can facilitate success in the rehabilitative process. In this chapter, a tool for analyzing personality types is described. Then specific examples are presented demonstrating how audiologists can use this information to augment the aural rehabilitation (including hearing aids) process.

FORMAL PERSONALITY TYPING IN AURAL REHABILITATION

The neopsychoanalytic work of Carl Jung (Jung, 1920), though controversial to some, offers a unique method of organizing personalities into specific types. Although we utilize many different theories in the process of working with our patients, Jung offered a specific method by which we can describe our patients' personal styles. This categorization greatly facilitates our capability to "tune" the rehabilitative process to the patient, rather than treating all patients the same.

Myers-Briggs Type Indicator®

In 1942, inspired by the recently translated work of Carl Jung, Katherine Briggs and her daughter, Isabel Myers, began experimenting with an evaluation of personal characteristics that could differentiate one personality from another. Motivated by their conviction that World War II was caused, in part, by people not understanding differences, and observing extreme variations between Isabel and her husband, they evaluated all their family members, the people their children dated, and many others to determine their psychological types. Published as a theoretical construct in 1943 (Briggs & Myers, 1943, 1976), the Myers Briggs Type Indicator (MBTI®) was later published as a psychological tool in 1956 by the Education Testing Service. By the 1960s the MBTI was considered to be a valid measurement of personality and reliable in reporting these personality differences over time. Currently, it is one of the most utilized assessment tools of personality for career counseling and motivational uses worldwide. The MBTI provides audiologists with a method of viewing how patients react to things, situations, and other people and presents opportunities for using this information in the rehabilitative treatment process. We can determine if our patients are outward or inward directed, move from one project to another, give up easily, are bothered by minor details, or are generally "laid back."

Classifying personality characteristics of patients who are hearing impaired is not a new concept. Staab (1985) described how patients react differently to hearing aids and offered a number of different types of patients (e.g., the "Engineer Type," the "High E Type"[extrovert], and the "High I Type"[introvert]). Each of these types produces certain clinical rehabilitative treatment challenges. A limitation of Staab's system was that he offered no real method of assessment to facilitate knowledge of personal style before patients are seen in the clinic, but simply offered possible explanations for various clinical situations.

The use of the Myers-Briggs Type Indicator (Myers, Kirby, & Myers,1993) has been suggested recently (Traynor & Buckles, 1996; Traynor, 1997, 1998) for use in audiology clinics. The MBTI identifies 16

Myers-Briggs Type Indicator and MBTI are registered trademarks of Consulting Psychologists Press, Inc.

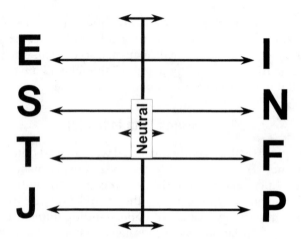

Figure 3–1. MBTI preference continuums.

distinctively different patterns describing how people interface with their instincts. These Jungian instincts or motivations, purposes, aims, values, drives, impulses, and urges create fundamental personality differences among people. Personal preference for a particular function is characteristic of how a person interfaces with these instincts, and thus, individuals may be typed by their preferences. Based on Jungian and probably other psychological theories, the MBTI uses personal situations and reactions to word pairs, adjusted by gender, to facilitate scores on four continuums. These four continuums consist of opposite scales of **Extraversion (E)/Introversion (I), Sensing (S)/Intuition (N), Thinking (T)/Feeling (F),** and **Judging (J)/Perceiving (P)** as shown in Figure 3–1. The scores on these four continuums make up the 16 personality types offered by the MBTI. For example, if a person scores toward the E side of the first continuum and the N side of the second, the F side of the third, and the J side on the fourth, his personality would be scored as an ENFJ.

Extraversion (E)/Introversion (I) Scale

Jung looked on *Extraversion* and *Introversion* as valuable opposites, utilized by everyone, but not in the same manner or with equal ease. Broadway (1964) indicated that 75% of the general population are *Extraverts* (E); they attune to the external environment and tend to be more interested and comfortable when they are working actively with people or things. *Extraverted* people prefer to communicate by conversation, often speaking first and reflecting later, and learn best by doing or discussing.

Introverts (I), however, make up 25% of the population and are drawn into an inner world, preferring to communicate by writing, and reflect before acting or speaking. *Introverts* learn best by reflection or mental exercise and are more comfortable when their work involves ideas. *Introverts* require a good deal of their activity to take place quietly inside their heads.

The main word that differentiates an *Extravert* from an *Introvert* is sociability as opposed to territoriality, but the extravert also finds breadth appealing, where the *Introvert* finds the notion of depth more attractive. Other notions that give cue to this continuum are the concepts: intensive interaction as opposed to concentration, multiplicity of relationships as opposed to limited relationships, expenditure of energy as opposed to conservation of energy, and interest in external happenings as opposed to interest in internal reactions.

Sensing (S)/Intuition (N) Scale

Jung believed there are two strategies utilized to find answers to problems or situations, *Sensing* or *Intuition (iNtuition)*. Sensing strategies use the eyes, ears, and other senses to tell what is actually occurring. The opposite strategy, *iNtuition*, uses meanings, relationships, and possibilities that are beyond the reach of the senses for fact gathering and is especially useful for seeing what might be done about a situation. One of these strategies is often preferred over the other. As the strategy is used, the individual attains more skills, becoming an expert at noticing all the observable facts, *Sensing* (S), or seeing a new possibility or solution, *iNtuition* (N).

Individuals tending to use the Sensing strategy typically become more realistic, practical, observant, fun loving, and good at remembering and working with a great number of facts. Those preferring *iNtuition* value imagination and inspiration and are creative in projects and problem solving.

Broadway (1964) indicated that 75% of the population utilize the sensing type strategy, while 25% use *iNtuition* (N). Careful listening to one's own choice of words may demonstrate how people verbalize their preferences. Through choice of vocabulary and intonation, one often transmits one value over another. People who prefer *Sensing* (S), for example, tend to value experience and the wisdom of the past and want to be realistic, whereas those who prefer *iNtuition* (N) tend to value hunches and a vision of the future and are likely to be speculative. Words such as actual, down-to-earth, no nonsense, fact, practical, and sensible are music to the ears of *Sensing* people. Words such as possible, fascinating, fantasy, fiction, ingenious, and imaginative are apt to light up the eyes of *iNtuition* people.

Thinking (T)/Feeling (F) Scale

The *Thinking* strategy, utilized by 50% of the population, predicts the logical result of any particular action by deciding impersonally on the basis of cause and effect, similar to the methods utilized by a computer. The opposite of this mechanical form of decision strategy is *Feeling*, used by the other 50% of the population. *Feeling* uses personal values and gives weight to anything that matters or is important to the individual or others in the decision, without requiring that it be logical.

In decision making, both *Thinking* and *Feeling* are utilized with equal confidence, but not simultaneously. Personalities that trust *thinking* more than *feeling* grow skillful at dealing with the world logically without the intervention of predictable human reactions. Those that trust *feeling* may be better at dealing with people. They are typically more sympathetic, appreciative, and tactful and give great weight to the personal values of themselves and others.

Impersonal choice people, the *Thinkers*, tend to respond positively to such words as objective, principles, policy, laws, criteria, firmness, justice, categories, standards, critique, analysis, and allocation. *Feelers* tend to react positively to words such as subjective, values, social values, extenuating circumstances, intimacy, persuasion, humane, harmony, good or bad, appreciate, sympathy, and devotion.

Persons scoring more toward the T side of the continuum tend to give priority to objective criteria, and are apt to be good at argumentation, attempting to win people over to their point of view through logic rather than appealing to emotions. Persons on the F side of the continuum tend to be good at persuasion and make choices in the context of the personal impact of the decision on others.

Perception (P)/Judgment (J) Scale

The last of the four continuums concerns *Judgment* and *Perception*. This continuum describes how a person relates to the outside world by choosing to use judging skills or perceiving skills. Fifty percent of the population are *Judgers* who use their judging process (the *Thinking-Feeling* continuum) to live in a planned, orderly way, in an effort to regulate and control their lives. Individuals who prefer a judging lifestyle tend to be scheduled, organized, systematic, and methodological. At the other end of the continuum are the 50% of the population who typically prefer to rely on a perceptive process (the *Sensing-iNtuition* continuum) for dealing with the outer world. *Perceivers* live in a spontaneous world, seeking to understand life and adapt to it. Individuals who prefer the *Perceiving* end of the continuum tend to be spontaneous, casual, and flexible, and prefer to have things loose and open-ended.

Judging people prefer words such as settled, decided, fixed, plan ahead, run one's life, closure, decision making, planned, completed, decisive, "wrap it up," urgency, deadlines, and "get the show on the road." Conversely, *Perceiving* people prefer expressions such as pending, gather more data, flexible, adapt as you go, let life happen, keep options open, "treasure hunting," open-ended, emergent, tentative, "something will happen," "there's plenty of time," "what deadline?," and "let's wait and see."

Obtaining MBTI Test Materials

In 1996, the official version of the MBTI consisted of 126 questions, and the only requirement to obtain the test materials and the software needed to score the MBTI was that professionals using it had a college level "Tests and Measurements" course as a component of their academic curriculum. Administering the official MBTI tests required about 20 minutes, and the subject had to have at least an eighth-grade reading level. The official MBTI scoring software, booklets, answer sheets, and so forth were available through psychological test material suppliers, such as Consulting Psychologists, Inc., Palo Alto, California (http://www.MBTI.com).

Currently, there is a less expensive, similar test available from Virtual Knowledge, Needham, MA (http://www.virtualknowledge.com). The materials contain a computer program that generates a 50-question test (Dean, 1997). The software actually presents the test and adjusts the number of questions according to the patient's answers. This program is used to administer and score the test, and the results are stored for statistical purposes and may be accessed at a later time. This software also provides an orientation to the Keirsian Temperament view (to be explained shortly) as well as the test; it is easy to administer, requires little memory, and costs about $25.00. Although it is not the MBTI, it is quite accurate (albeit a bit extreme on scale scores at times compared to the traditional MBTI) and facilitates patient care in a short amount of time.

Putting the MBTI Together

Once the MBTI is completed, the scores are generated on the various continua as presented in Figure 3–1. These scores are recorded on the basis of which side of the continuum the person's score resides, (i.e., closer to E than I, closer to S than to N, etc.). Thus, people who score in the areas that correspond to E, S, T, and J would be presented as a personal style of ESTJ, whereas those scoring in areas corresponding to I, N, F, and P would be presented as an INFP. In all there are 16 personal style types, each with its own set of characteristics, as summarized in Figure 3–2.

Keirsian Temperaments: A Personal Style Shorthand

It is possible to be overwhelmed considering eight extraverted types (ESTP, ESFP, ENTP, ENFP, ESTJ, ESFJ, ENFJ, ENTJ) and eight introverted types (ISTJ, ISFJ, INFJ, INTJ, ISTP, ISFP, INFP, INTP) that might be obtained on the MBTI. Kroeger and Thuesen (1988) indicated that there are several methods for looking at a type with a "personality shorthand" that can give clinicians specific keys to certain personal styles without having to concentrate on all of the traits at once. A common method for looking at these MBTI types is to take two letters (or traits) that many of these personality types have in common. This is called the Keirsian Temperament (KT). The foregoing two groups of eight types can then be divided into subgroups designated by two letters, symbolizing similar characteristics. For example, the ESTJ, ESFJ, ENFJ, and ENTJ could be organized together as EJs, whereas the INTJ, INFP, INFJ, and INFP types can be organized into INs. Similarly, the ISFP, INFP, ESFP, and ENFP could be considered as FPs. The manner in which individuals **gather information** is defined on the S-N continuum and constitutes the first letter of the KT. Typically, *Sensors* focus only on what is actually there, whereas *iNtuitors* are optimistic and see the possibilities. For the concept of seeing the forest through the trees, the *Sensor* sees a tree, the *iNtuitor* sees a forest. *Sensors* tend to be pessimistic and see the "cup as half empty," whereas the more optimistic *iNtuitor* sees the cup as half full. In KT, the first letter reflects how the person actually gathers information, thus it will always be either an S or an N.

The second important preference is how you prefer to evaluate the data you have gathered: objectively *(Thinking)* or subjectively *(Feeling)*. The second letter of the temperament is defined on the T-F continuum and is determined in part by the first letter. That is, if you are *iNtuitive* (N), your preference for gathering data is abstract and conceptual. Therefore two of the basic temperament groups are the **NF** and the **NT.** *Sensors* tend to gather their information by methods that are concrete and tactile. To *Sensors,* the next most important function is not how to evaluate the data, but what to do with the data: organize *(Judging)* or continue to collect or seek more *(Perceiving)*. Thus, the other two Keirsian Temperaments are SJ and SP. Kroeger and Thuesen (1988) offered

	Sensing Types		Intuitive Types	
Introversion	**ISTJ** Serious, Quiet, Practical, Logical, Matter of Fact, Dependable, Realistic, Take Responsibility	**ISFJ** Quiet, Friendly, Responsible, Thorough, Painstaking, Conscientious, Accurate, Concerned for Others	**INFJ** Succeed by Perseverance, Originality, Quietly Forceful, Conscientious, Principles, Concerned for Others	**INTJ** Original Minds, Great Drive, Long Range Vision, Organized, Skeptical, Critical, Independent, High Standards, Determined
	ISTP Quiet, Reserved, Observing, Mechanical, Cause/Effect, How and Why Things Work, Find Practical Solutions,	**ISFP** Retiring, Quietly Friendly, Sensitive, Kind, Modest, Shun Disagreements, Do not Force Their Opinions	**INFP** Quiet Observers, Idealistic, Loyal, Courteous, Adaptable, Flexible, Little Concern for Possessions or Surroundings	**INTP** Quiet and Reserved, Theoretical, Scientific Problem Solvers, Logical, No Small Talk, Sharply Defined Interests
Extraversion	**ESTP** On-the-Spot Problem Solvers, Focus on Getting Results, Dislike Long Explanations,	**ESFP** Outgoing, Accepting, Friendly, Enjoy Everything, Sound Common Sense, Likes Facts, not Theory	**ENFP** Warmly Enthusiastic, Distractible, Ingenious, Does not Plan Ahead, Rely on Ability to Improvise	**ENTP** Quick, Good at Many things, Stimulating Company, Alert, Finds Logical Reasons for What They Want, May Argue for Fun
	ESTJ Practical, Realistic, Decisive, Matter of Fact, Not Interested in Abstract concepts or Theories, Organizers	**ESFJ** Warm Hearted, Talkative, Popular, Conscientious, Need Encouragement and Praise, Need Harmony	**ENFJ** Responsible, Responsive, Responds to Praise and Criticism, Sociable, Popular, Sympathetic	**ENTJ** Frank, Decisive, Leaders in activities, Good at Reasoning, Enjoy adding to their knowledge, Likes to talk

Figure 3–2. MBTI personality types. (Reprinted with permission from *Introduction to Type* [5th Ed.], by I. Myers, L. K. Kirby, and K. D. Myers, 1993, p. XX. Palo Alto, CA: Consulting Psychologists Press, Inc.)

Table 3–1. Keirsian Temperaments and Associated MBTI Types.

NF		NT		SJ		SP	
ENFJ	INFJ	ENTJ	INTJ	ESTJ	ISTJ	ESFP	ISFP
ENFP	INFP	ENTP	INTP	ESFJ	ISFJ	ESTP	ISTP

that this is a behaviorally sound method of personality typing. Table 3–1 presents the organization of the KTs relative to the MBTI personal styles.

Although the MBTI can be useful to audiologists in their rehabilitative endeavors, the KTs offer some distinct, simpler possibilities as we work with patients on a day-to-day basis.

AURAL REHABILITATIVE USES OF TYPING

Figure 3–2 (Myers, 1962; Myers & Myers, 1980) presented the various MBTI personality types. Personality type appears to be a relatively uninvestigated variable of hearing impairment that could be utilized to describe how patients react to their hearing loss, hearing aids, loudness growth, recruitment, tinnitus, the isolation created by the impairment, and other known complications of a hearing deficit. These various personality types, predicted by either the full MBTI or the abbreviated KT shorthand, may react more favorably to certain rehabilitative management techniques. Audiologists' knowledge of patients' particular strategies for coping with their hearing deficits may allow them to choose more appropriate products and to individualize the rehabilitative process. The possibilities for the use of personal style as assessed by the MBTI in audiology are numerous. Consider that hearing impairment might be more "isolating" for an ENFP type than an INTJ type. Communicating is not a necessary basic need for INTJs; it is, however, basic and an intrinsic component for ENFPs because they are people oriented and require interaction with others to facilitate their needs for human interaction. Other personal style variables might include higher hearing aid expectations for an ESTJ than for an ISFP. Further, it *might* be possible (although there are no data to confirm this supposition) that the hearing aid return rate for INTJs would be higher than for patients exhibiting the ENFJs.

Earlier in this chapter it was suggested that two patients having similar audiometric configurations can react quite differently to their deficits. Could these different reactions to the same hearing impairment be quantified somewhat by MBTI personality type? Do some personality types react differently to reduced dynamic ranges or are, to some extent, reduced dynamic ranges a function of personality type? For example, is it possible that an ESFP type person is more sensitive to changes in loudness growth than an INTP? Is tinnitus more annoying for a person who is inwardly directed than for an outwardly directed person? Could it be that our current rehabilitative strategies are geared toward IN personality types that make up only 4% of the general population rather than to the EN personality type that is found 52% of the time (Myers et al. 1993)?

Establishing patients' personality styles can result in some logical modifications in counseling. For example, some personality types prefer concrete explanations of variables, products, and other rehabilitative concepts, whereas for others this information should be omitted. Some personality types prefer to know how many patients have used this product successfully; others want to hear the whole story about why the product worked, what particulars made this device work better than the competition, and how much better it performed.

ESTJ types respect the clinician's authority and seem to feel that "you are the Doctor," allowing you to do whatever you think is appropriate for their hearing impairment. They do, however, like to see things done correctly and are impatient with clinicians who, in their perception, do not carry out procedures with sufficient attention to detail in order to "get the job done right." The ESTJ is constantly evaluating the audiologist's clinical performance by the success of the procedures, products, and adjustments to the hearing aid.

Although an ESTJ patient does not typically require or want lengthy explanations of the principles and/or theories behind products, they are, however, interested in summaries of how these products have performed for your other patients. A common ESTJ question might be, "How many other people have this hearing aid?" or "Am I the only one with these problems?" Long discussions of circuitry, loudness growth, or other detailed concepts should probably be avoided with the ESTJ personality.

INTJs are not impressed with the clinician's research or publications, nor do they care how many speeches have been presented in the past or about those that will come in the future. This type usually requires extra time for clinicians to develop a good rationale for the proposed procedures and/or products. Once the rationale is developed to their satisfaction and it makes sense to them, they will adopt it. If, however, the rationale for the procedure is not explained well enough to gain their support, it will be rejected and products may be returned or the hearing aids may end up living in the dresser drawer. Because these patients trust their own insight and are not easily impressed by authority, the extra time spent discussing various types and styles of circuits for hearing aids and rationales for the specific tests conducted may be essential to gain full participation. Patients with an INTJ personal style love challenges, and once convinced about the strategy, will typically "stick with it," even if the procedure is not going well. INTJ personal styles abhor confusion, mess, and inefficiency; thus, clinically, these perceptions may cause extreme difficulties for success if patients believe that these factors exist in the rehabilitative intervention process.

Additionally, they are "team players" who respond very well to the concept of "being on a team" in the rehabilitative process with the clinician and others including spouses, family members, and friends. Although INTJs assess everything with a critical eye, they will participate as long as they understand everything that is being done for them.

Informal Use of Personality Typing

It is not always practical to conduct a formal assessment of personality type. In this case, it is important to conduct at least an informal assessment of personality type in order to determine some of the generic needs of patients. Traditionally, experienced audiologists actually do this quite often by comparing the current patient to ones seen last week or last month.

A general determination of type may often be accomplished by conducting small talk or dialog during the case history. Further, when these responses are combined with observations, type estimates may be quite accurate.

Informally Observable J-P Differences

The easiest of all to assess informally are the *Judging-Perceiving* (J-P) differences. Judgers tend to remain more focused on a task or topic, whereas *Perceivers* tend to move easily from one topic to another, sometimes seeming scattered. *Judgers* have a built-in time clock, and *Perceivers* have no innate sense of schedule. *Perceivers* tend to generate alternatives to any situation, whereas *Judgers* tend to get locked up in one method. While *Judgers* offer decisive opinions on most topics, *Perceivers* are less likely to do so, often preferring to answer a question with a question.

In aural rehabilitation, *Judgers* are the patients who have made up their mind on the type and style of hearing instruments they want and often have decided how many they need even before the clinician has had a discussion with them. *Judging* patients may require minimal clinical time. For example, the patient may come into the clinic and want to purchase a single brand X hearing aid because he has just known too many friends that did not do very well with two. Conversely, some *Judgers* require extra time because they have not yet formed a firm opinion. They need to listen to the audiologist present detailed information about the various types, styles, and technologies that are the most appropriate. These patients actually need **all** the information available, and possibly some discussion about how these products work, to facilitate their decision. Once the decision is made, *Judgers* will carry it through as a substantial commitment because they tend to "just know they are right." Further, with sensitivity for time, they will be appreciative of the extra time taken with them.

Perceivers, however, are the patients who seem never to be able to make up their minds with questions such as, "What if hearing aids get better, shouldn't I wait?" These patients have actual difficulty with closure and feel that they have to consider new information constantly. Further, these patients have some difficulty with deadlines and other time constraints, tending to use extra clinic time for that one last question. The following is an example of a dialogue with a *Judging* patient.

Clinician: What can I do for you today?

Patient: I've decided that I need a brand X hearing aid for my right ear. My left ear is OK for now. My friends all have brand X and it is the best, so that's what I want. Oh yes, I want one of those little tiny hearing aids that go so far in your ear that you can't see it.

Clinician: Well, what we need to do is a hearing evaluation and then discuss the type and style of amplification that will best suit your needs.

Patient: I won't buy one of those "expensive" hearing aids, because I know that all hearing aids are the same inside, with only just a different name on the outside.

Clinician: Although it was often true that conventional hearing aids were similar a few years ago, there are now some proprietary hearing aid circuits that truly make major differences in performance. There are studies that confirm these circuitry differences and their benefits. Often these more "expensive" circuits are very much worth their extra cost.

Continued

Patient: I have two friends who have used brand X and that's what I need too! I don't really have that much of a hearing loss anyway. Well, let's get to it; I don't want to take up too much of your time today.

Judging patients have often made up their minds about what they need and will tell clinicians what they feel will meet their needs. The capability to change according to the professional recommendation will depend on the other characteristics of their personality.

This may also be relevant to patients who feel they do not have a hearing loss and have decided not to do anything about it. Often the reason they are in the clinic is to please a friend or relative (i.e., "My wife thinks I have a hearing loss"). These patients can be a formidable clinical challenge as well, and clinical success will depend on how the evidence of the impairment is presented and the patients' other personality characteristics. *Judgers* have usually made up their minds about what their needs are for a particular item, such as amplification. Once decisions are made, no matter if based on solid or erroneous data, it will require the patients' other characteristics to facilitate modifications in their decisions. The following is a sample of a dialogue with a *Perceiving* patient.

Clinician: What are we doing for you today?

Patient: Well, I'm here to see if I have a hearing loss. My daughter says that she thinks I don't hear well. I have had this appointment scheduled a couple of times before, but always something "came up." What's that picture on the wall?

Clinician: That's a picture of the anatomy of the ear.

Patient: Boy, there sure is a lot inside the ear! My daughter thinks that I turn up the TV too loud and I don't really think so. Say, that is a nice bright shirt you're wearing! I just can't wear that color at all.

Clinician: What we need to do is conduct a hearing evaluation and then discuss the results to see if you do have a hearing impairment.

Patient: I don't need a hearing aid to talk to you; do you think that I *really* need hearing aids?

Clinician: That's what we'll find out from the hearing evaluation.

Perceivers are easily distracted and often have difficulty focusing on the particular problem at hand. Clinicians need to bring them back to the topic and focus on various issues, ensuring that they understand each one. *Perceivers* generally do not have a good sense of time, and these minor distractions can waste a great deal of clinic time. Clinicians need to keep these patients "on track" and focused on the hearing rehabilitative techniques being conducted. There is nothing worse for the clinic schedule than a whole day of *Perceiving* patients, because it is difficult to stay on time for the next appointment.

Perceivers often cannot handle a presentation of all of the amplification options, because they have too much difficulty focusing on a specific item. It is necessary to summarize the information for them.

Informally Observable E-I Differences

Another obvious difference to the informal observer is the *Extraversion-Introversion* (E-I). Typically, *Extraverts* speak more enthusiastically, rapidly, and loudly than introverts. In fact, the *Introvert* sometimes wants to "hush" the *Extraverts*. *Introverts* may feel as if they are drained by conversations. They tend to think before they speak, usually understating their point, whereas *Extraverts* overstate things and repeat themselves. Further, *Extraverts* also use more nonverbal communication such as hand waving, facial movements, and so forth, whereas *Introverts* may be more aloof and reserved in these mannerisms.

In addition to the differences in "outgoingness," another easily observable factor in the informal assessment of type relative to *Extraverts* and *Introverts* is the different level of energy for conversation. *Extraverts* tend to increase their energy level and enthusiasm for the conversation as it continues. *Introverts* tend to reduce their energy.

Extraverts are relatively easy to interact with clinically. They freely, sometimes too freely, present their case history and readily answer questions. It must be realized that they tend to verbalize their thinking or "think out loud" by presenting ideas and refining them as they speak. These patients will often keep talking as long as you are willing to listen, and clinicians must watch the time carefully. Some situations may even require statements such as " Today, I did not allow time for that," "We must have another appointment," or "We will take care of that at your next appointment."

Introverts are different in that they need time to reflect before responding. Depending on the degree of *Introversion,* it can be quite difficult to obtain case histories and ascertain enough information about these patients to make intelligent clinical decisions about rehabilitative problems until they "let you know them."

The following is a sample dialogue with an Extraverted patient.

Clinician: Good morning Sir, How is it going?

Patient: Fine. My daughter brought me to the clinic today, and we had a great breakfast over at that new restaurant on Tenth Avenue. Do you know the place?

Clinician: Yes, I know the place, but I haven't been there yet. Is it any good?

Patient: Oh, it's just very good. I had the ham and cheese omelet, and their coffee is the best!

Clinician: Well, what brings you to see me today?

Patient: Well, my wife and daughter think I have a hearing loss. I haven't heard very well for some time now, and I suppose that I need hearing aids as I am getting older. I have some difficulty with conversations, and I'm turning the TV up these days. Actually, I don't think I have much trouble. So I guess that we'll find out this morning.

Clinician: Well, let's go over your history.

Patient: OK, well it's been about 4 to 5 years now, and it seems to be worse on the right side because when I lay on my left side I can't hear as well as when I lay on my right side. I can't hear as well on the phone on the right ear either. I don't know, maybe it is wax in there—you know, sometimes I get a little bit out of there on my Q-tips. What causes that wax anyway?

Clinician: We'll get to the wax in a minute, but now let's focus on your history. So, do you have any ringing or buzzing noises in your head?

Patient: Oh do I ever! My ears both ring all the time. There is this little high-pitched noise that constantly goes "Rinnnnnnnnng" all the time. It used to drive me nuts, but I'm used to it now. It's actually a bit louder in the right ear.

Clinician: Have you worked around loud noise?

Patient: All my life. I started as a kid on the farm on them old tractors, the John Deere ones, they made a "PoPing" sound. You know that you could get about 10 more horsepower from them old ones if you took the mufflers off. Well, anyway I left the farm to go to World War II, and I was in the artillery. Those loud guns got me, I think. Of course, then I went on to work for the packing company, and you know that's awful loud, too.

The same conversation with an *Introverted* patient is quite different as illustrated in the following example.

Clinician: Good morning, sir, how is it going today?

Patient: Fine.

Clinician: What brings you to see me today?

Patient: I think I may need hearing aids.

Clinician: Well, sir, let's go over your history.

Patient: [No response]

Clinician: How long have you had this hearing loss?

Patient: Last 4 to 5 years.

Clinician: Is one ear better than the other?

Patient: Left.

Clinician: Do you have any ringing or buzzing noises in your head?

Patient: Yes.

Clinician: What does it sound like?

Patient: Ringing.

Clinician: High-pitched or low-pitched ringing?

Patient: High.

Clinician: Have you worked around loud noise during your career?

Patient: Yes.

Clinician: What kind of loud noise did you work around?

Patient: Tractors.

With these patients, we need to "extract" the information from them to facilitate the examination and recommendation of the hearing instrument.

Informally Observable S-N Differences

Compared to the J-P and E-I differences, the *Sensing-iNtuitive* preference is more difficult to observe informally because it is not readily observable in the form of words or actions. Patients presenting an *iNtuitive* nature tend to look for the meaning of an event or an experience, whereas *Sensors* examine the specific components of the experience. For example, *Sensors* might focus on all of the hearing that is lost, but *iNtuitives* would focus on the amount of residual hearing and what can still be done with what remains. Further, *Sensors* might focus on all of the things wrong with a hearing aid, whereas *iNtuitives* might focus on the good experiences or positive things about the device. The following is a sample dialogue with a *Sensing* patient.

Clinician: So, how did your new hearing aids work for you?

Patient: Well, I don't like them, but I know that I need them. I have a sore spot in my left ear, here by the part of my ear where it's indented, and it's OK on the right. I couldn't hear at Rotary Club or in church. When I got to Rotary, I sat close to the speaker and I couldn't hear the guy next to me. We had a group sitting around in a circle telling jokes, and I had some trouble getting the punch lines. At church, I couldn't hear the minister in my usual seat, and when the music started, I thought I would be knocked out of my seat! I seem to have more difficulty with women's voices and with the wrinkling of paper. My own voice sounds strange to me as well.

Clinician: Did you do OK with your wife's voice and with the television, and were you able to hear the grandchildren?

Patient: Yes, I seem to do very well in those situations.

Clinician: Let's take these situations one at a time. First, we'll modify the left device so it fits you better, then make some program changes that will, hopefully, improve your performance and eliminate your sensitivity to loud music. We'll want to see you again in about 10 days to determine how these changes have affected the instrument's performance.

Notice that *Sensing* patients focus on the things that are wrong with the instruments, rather than focusing on the situations where they provide benefit. Obtaining information regarding the patient's benefit is usually a more difficult task, and it must be, at times, extracted from Sensing patients. Now note the sample dialogue with the *iNtuitive* patient.

Clinician: So, how did your new hearing aids work for you?

Patient: Well, I can hear my wife a lot better. Although they may be a bit loud, I can hear my grandchildren, and the television is comfortable for me at levels that are comfortable for others. I guess I'll get used to the extra loudness in time. The hearing aids really work, that's for sure.

Clinician: What specific difficulties did you encounter during the time you tried the hearing aids?

Patient: Well, my voice sounds different, but I could probably get used to that. I have a problem in group situations and at church. I have a sore spot in my ear on the right, but it's OK on the left.

Clinician: Tell me a bit more about the situations where you had difficulty.

Patient: I couldn't hear at Rotary Club or in church. When I got to Rotary, I sat close to the speaker and I could not hear the guy next to me. We had a group sitting around in a circle telling jokes and I had some trouble getting the punch lines. At church, I couldn't hear the minister in my usual seat, and when the music started, it was really annoying! I seem to have more difficulty with women's voices and with the wrinkling of paper, but again, I think it will take me a little while to adapt.

Clinician: Let's take these situations one at a time. We'll modify the right device so that it fits you better, then we'll make some program changes that will assist your performance with the device. We'll want to see you again in about 10 days to determine how these changes have affected your performance with the instruments.

The *iNtuitors* may require more extraction of information from the negative side, whereas the *Sensors* may have difficulty realizing benefit. It is obvious that these patients are saying the same things in these dialogues, but focusing on different aspects of their performance with the devices. The clinical adjustments are the same; it is simply the patients' focus that is different. So, proper counseling becomes critically important. Clinically, with *Sensors* it is a hasty decision; they are not happy with the hearing aids. With *iNtuitors,* they may not be entirely satisfied with the devices, but they hesitate to say so because they hold on for the promise that real benefit will take some time. It is necessary to probe *iNtuitors* with questions to investigate possible problems, whereas "handholding" *Sensors* may be necessary to reassure them.

Informally Observable T-F Differences

Because the *Thinking-Feeling* continuum involves the decision-making process, it is often very difficult to observe informally in the clinic. This T-F process involves how patients critique, evaluate, and decide about the information they have gathered through their *Sensing* and *iNtuition* systems. Thus, *Thinking-Feeling* assessments are the most difficult of all personality traits to observe clinically. Although both types of patients have feelings, *Feelers* want to experience their feelings, whereas *Thinkers* prefer to understand them. Generally, *Thinkers* are capable of looking at situations objectively, often making statements that may sound a bit uncaring and unfeeling to others. *Feelers,* however, are pleaser-type individuals who seek harmony in all their relationships, no matter with whom. They feel an intense need, and sometimes even a responsibility, to ensure that fairness and others' feelings are considered at all costs. It is difficult to plan clinic time for either *Thinkers* or *Feelers,* because they may make decisions based on their rationales either immediately (*Thinkers*) or after lengthy discussion (*Feelers*).

Thinkers tend to look at the cause and effect of a situation (e.g., "I have a hearing impairment; therefore, I need hearing aids."). Indeed, these individuals can be counseled with objective information, such as the audiogram. Further, various situations can be discussed where the impairment has created difficulty for them. Once they are convinced there is really a hearing deficit, *Thinkers* will logically conclude there is reason to consider products essential to the rehabilitative process. A similar reasonable and logical presentation of the rationale for the use of specific hearing products and application of the various technologies will usually result in a positive patient response. *Thinkers* make decisions based on the logical interpretation of information without consideration for the feelings of others, such as those who need to communicate with them. *Thinkers* respond well to detailed explanations of audiometric results and logical application of techniques to facilitate rehabilitative intervention.

Correspondingly, *Feelers* respond to discussions about how difficult it is for others to communicate with them or how their grandchildren may want to interact with them. Concentration on the ability to communicate with others will be important in their decision-making process. It is imperative to "touch their hearts" in rehabilitative techniques by involving family members or friends when explaining product technology or when instructing patients regarding the use of the instruments. The following is a sample dialogue with a *Thinking* patient.

Clinician: Now that we have discussed your hearing impairment and concluded that hearing instruments are the treatment for your hearing loss, it's necessary for us to discuss the devices themselves.

Patient: I noticed that you said *devices;* can't I get by with just one?

Clinician: Although you probably hear better with a single hearing aid than with none at all, you'll be able to optimize your hearing ability with hearing aids for each ear. Your depth perception of sound will be much better.

Patient: What do you mean by depth perception of sound?

Clinician: Sound will stand out better with amplification provided for both ears. Just as one sees better with a "monocle," it is still difficult to tell if one object is closer than another. When visual correction is provided for both eyes, however, depth perception is maintained as well as the capability to read in difficult lighting conditions. Hearing is somewhat the same in that when amplification is provided for both ears, certain auditory sounds stand out from other sounds. Further, distance hearing is better, and one is able to tell more easily from which direction sound is coming.

Patient: OK, so I understand that you are recommending that I buy hearing aids for both ears?

Clinician: Yes.

Patient: I've been told that these hearing aids are very expensive, but there is only about $85.00 worth of parts in those things.

Clinician: The parts of a hearing aid represent only a fraction of its cost [*the reader is referred to Chapter 4 for a more complete lay*
Continued

explanation of this issue]. Someone has to design the circuit and custom build the instrument according to your ear. The device then needs to be fit according to a prescription for your hearing loss and adjusted as necessary, depending on your lifestyle. The manufacturer and I both warrant the instrument to you for at least 1 year. When you think about it, a hearing aid is much more than just the parts.

Patient: What kind of hearing aids should I get? Do I have to have those big ones that go behind my ear? I sure don't want something that big and obvious, unless of course, I really have to.

The remainder of the session would typically involve a detailed description of the different styles of hearing aids, specifics on hearing aid technology and how these products typically perform under various listening conditions. *Thinking* patients not only require a full explanation of the products currently on the market, but also the principles and procedures involved in the provision of rehabilitative treatment. These patients require discussion as to **why** the clinician has used a particular method, style, or hearing aid technology. These discussions can become quite lengthy, but are essential to obtaining the confidence and cooperation of the patient in the rehabilitative process. Without these discussions, *Thinking* patients will not have the understanding necessary to feel comfortable with the various procedures and products. Contrast the previous dialogue with the following one for a *Feeling* patient.

Clinician: Let's discuss your hearing evaluation and the ramifications of what we have found.

Patient: OK.

Clinician [*using the audiogram as a counseling tool*]: As you can see, this graph represents your hearing impairment. The numbers on the top represent the pitch of the sound from low pitches to high pitches, and the numbers along the side refer to loudness. The line on the graph represents how loud I needed to adjust each sound so that you could just barely hear it.

Patient: OK, I see that.

Clinician: Have people indicated that you are not hearing as well now as in the past?

Patient: Oh, I know I don't hear as well as I used to because I've been missing parts of conversations for quite awhile now. My family complains a lot and that bothers me. They think I don't care about what they're saying, but I do. I just don't know if hearing aids will help this problem

Clinician: Hearing aids would definitely help you hear better and make it much easier for them to communicate with you. You see, with your hearing impairment you can't hear the high pitches as well as the low pitches. This makes it especially difficult to understand high-frequency voices, such as children and women.

To motivate *Feeling* patients, it is essential that they feel that others are affected by their hearing impairment. The decision to proceed in the rehabilitative process will be determined by how much of their life is disrupted by their hearing impairment. Because they are sensitive to the needs of others, explanations should emphasize their abilities to communicate with others and how the treatment program or products will make life better or easier for those around them.

Effect of Clinician's Personal Style

The personal style of the clinician may also make a substantial difference in the degree of successful patient interaction. Personal style may explain why certain patients do better with some clinicians than with others or why some clinicians become frustrated with certain types of patients. Think of the type of patient who causes you to be frustrated or angry. For example, some clinicians have much difficulty with patients who "talk your leg off," whereas others actually enjoy these patients. The INTJ type of clinician is not comfortable with lots of dialogue and is interested in moving the situation along to achieve results, whereas the ENFJ clinician is more comfortable with patients who need to talk about how they feel when they talk with their grandchildren and so forth.

It is possible that the patient types that are the furthest from our own present the most clinical challenge. For example, a clinician who is an ENFJ might have the most difficulty with a patient who is an ISTP. Clinicians must learn to work with the opposites to their own particular personality. *Extraverted* clinicians must extract information from *Introverted* patients. *iNtuitive* clinicians who have constructed positive blueprints for rehabilitative plans may need to deal with *Sensing* patients who have more pessimistic attitudes toward the process. *Feeling* clinicians may worry about how patients are emotionally dealing with friends and relatives, whereas *Thinking* clinicians may focus solely on the hearing of patients. Finally, *Judging* clinicians may find it difficult and extremely frustrating to deal with *Perceiving* patients who jump from topic to topic.

Although it is impossible for us to change our personality totally for the clinic, it is possible to reduce the adverse affects. For example, *Introverted* clinicians must make an effort to be especially outgoing and interactive, and *Thinking* clinicians should attempt to present the *Feeling* arguments for various situations and so forth. Understanding one's own personality and the advantages and limitations when interacting with certain types of patients can be a major asset to clinical success. For the patients who present extremely difficult interactions for certain clinicians, it may be necessary to schedule them with another clinician to provide the best possible rehabilitative care.

SUMMARY

The following outline summarizes the important concepts of this chapter.

iNtuitive/Feeling Types (NF)
Typical NF patient will ask you

1. What are my rehabilitative options?
2. What are some possible experimental options that have real possibilities?
3. How will this affect all of the people concerned?

NF patients

Will let others influence their decisions.

Will think a lot before they act on a rehabilitative action.

iNtutive/Thinking Types (NT)
Typical NT patient will ask you

1. What are the pros and cons of this particular instrument and/or rehabilitative plan?
2. What is the logical outcome of each of these rehabilitative options?
3. Why has this option worked so well in the past?
4. What is the newest technology and tell me why it's better than the old technology?

NT Patients

Are concerned with the consequences of not acting to do something.

Tend to be firm minded.

Are not impressed by your credentials.

May expect you to explain the impairment, your rationale for the rehabilitative plan, and the rehabilitative plan in detail.

Sensing/ Perceiving Types (SP)
Typical SP patient will ask you:

1. What are the facts?
2. What instruments and philosophies have been successful for others with their hearing loss?
3. What are your opinions on their hearing difficulties?

SP patients

Learn best through experience.

Do not like restrictive situations.

Tend to postpone decisions while searching for options.

Sensing/Judging Types (SJ)
Typical SJ patient will ask you

1. What are the "bottom-line" realities of my hearing loss?
2. What are the specifics of the situation?
3. What have other patients with their hearing impairment done for this problem?

SJ patients

Tend to be very receptive to suggestions from authority figures.

Are impressed by your credentials.

Like to get things settled and finished.

Tend to be satisfied once a decision is made.

This chapter provides a rationale for assessing personality type as a basis for hearing rehabilitative treatment. Though the assessment may be conducted formally, most of the time it must be done informally as part of the overall rehabilitative intervention process. Professionals are in the beginning stages of using this technique to improve patient interactions, not only in Audiology but in other fields as well. Although this technique holds much promise, further research is warranted to understand fully the benefits of using personality type in the development of treatment schemes.

REFERENCES

Briggs, K. C., & Myers, I. B. (1943, 1976). *Myers-Briggs Type Indicator.* Palo Alto, CA: Consulting Psychologists Press.

Broadway, K. (1964). Jung's psychological types. *Journal of Analytical Psychology, 9,* 29–135.

Dean, D. H. (1997). *Personality test* [Computer software]. Needham, MA: Virtual Knowledge, Inc.

Jung, C. G. (1920). *Psychological types.* Princeton, NJ: Princeton University Press, Inc.

Keirsey, D., & Bates, M. (1984). *Please understand me.* Del Mar, CA: Gnosology Books, Ltd.

Kroeger, O., & Theusen, J. M. (1988). *Type talk.* New York: Dell Publishing

Myers, I. (1962) *Manual for the Myers-Briggs Type Indicator.* Palo Alto, CA: Consulting Psychologists Press, Inc.

Myers, I., Kirby, L. K., & Myers, K. D. (1993). *Introduction to Type (5th ed.).* Palo Alto, CA: Consulting Psychologists Press, Inc.

Myers, I., & Myers, P. (1980). *Gifts differing.* Palo Alto, CA: Consulting Psychologists Press, Inc.

Staab, W. (1985). *Types of hearing impaired patients.* Presentation at the Jackson Hole Rendezvous, Jackson Hole, Wyoming.

Traynor, R. M. (1998, April). *Personal style: The key to patient focused hearing care.* Paper presented at the annual meeting of the American Academy of Audiology, Los Angeles, CA.

Traynor, R. M., & Buckles, K. M. (1996). Personality typing: Audiology's new crystal ball. In S. Kochkin (Ed.), High performance hearing solutions (Vol. I). *Monograph to Hearing Review,* pp. 32–38.

Traynor, R. M., & Buckles, K. M. (1997, April). *Personal style: Patient focused aural rehabilitation.* Paper presented at the annual meeting of the American Academy of Audiology, Ft. Lauderdale, FL.

In Chapters 2 and 3, the importance of gathering information from and about patients was emphasized. Communication is a two-way street. However, a vital component of the counseling process is providing education. As we all recall from school, there are teachers who have the ability to get their points across in a clear and meaningful fashion, and there are others who, despite their knowledge, are unable or unwilling to pass their wisdom along to their students. However, it would be unfair to place all the blame for communication breakdowns on the message content and style of the teacher. Instead, it may be the student who is not comprehending information, and who, without a means of informing the teacher that he does not understand, further sinks into a quagmire. Also, some students are more intelligent than others, some are more interested in the subject, and some have experience they can build on. Teachers must present information in a manner that is concise, clear, relevant, and, most important, understandable to students. Similarly, hearing specialists must educate patients so that they not only understand the role hearing aids play as part of the rehabilitative process, but so that they can also discuss them with their professionals and the process can progress in a positive direction. In Chapter 4, Lori Pakulski considers the important matter of how to convey relevant information to patients, recognizing the vast differences among learning styles and levels of sophistication among patients. Much of the information contained in the sample boxes can be adapted for handouts and newsletters in your practice.

4

Conveying Information to Patients

■ Lori Pakulski, Ph.D. ■

Advanced hearing instrument technology has compelled dispensing audiologists to increase their knowledge and develop a new set of skills in order to evaluate and dispense products as well as counsel patients. Concurrently, the information explosion has produced a generation of more inquisitive, educated, and demanding consumers. Not all patients, however, are or should be assumed to be sophisticated and knowledgeable about hearing loss and amplification. Therefore, conveying accurate information to patients has taken on increased importance.

METHODS OF INSTRUCTING PATIENTS

As students and then professionals, we learn complex ideas and technical explanations about the auditory system, hearing aids, and audiological assessment. It is our job to translate technical language into meaningful information for our patients. The more appropriately educated the patients, the more likely they will succeed. As new developments and studies emerge, it becomes increasingly difficult to provide our patients with an understandable explanation of technical issues.

Because each patient has different skills and experiences, education, and preconceived notions, our task requires much consideration.

Recognizing certain characteristics of a patient's learning process may augment the manner in which information about hearing aids is conveyed. Aspects of personality assessment were discussed in Chapter 3. The following informal procedures can be used to obtain information about patients' learning strategies to optimize the educational process.

- Observe patients in the waiting room.

    Place audiologic/hearing aid-related brochures for patient reading. What type of literature attracts the patient's interest? If the patient reads this "scientific" type of material, you may be dealing with a person who will desire detailed explanations of technology.

    If possible, have a consumer-appropriate video playing in the waiting room. As you take patients back for services, inquire about the information they gleaned from the video. Visual learners, motivated to learn about their hearing health care, will likely have picked up some valuable information and may have questions.

- Evaluate the case history. How neat and complete are the forms? Patients who type or neatly print the information in a very thorough manner (often referring to old medical or audiological reports for supporting information) might suggest that they appreciate detailed information presented in a straightforward manner. Conversely, patients who supply only cursory information and instead spend time inquiring about how many patients with the same problem are seen, may be better served by at least initially limiting instruction to concrete facts and necessary discussion.
- Often, patients who are technologically oriented will arrive with their "homework" done. This type of patient reads reports on hearing aids from the Internet or *Consumer's Reports.* They may even contact companies to get information about certain products. These patients may benefit from explanations of studies they have read or from discussions about misconceptions they may have developed. Other patients may prefer that you provide them with "the bottom-line" and just get started. In either case, when discussions regarding technical issues arise, it is important to quiz patients in a nonthreatening manner to determine their knowledge levels.
- As discussed in Chapter 2, body language cues can also provide much information. Observe if the patient leans in (showing interest)

or backs away (seeming distracted). Does the patient actively take part in the conversation or hands-on practice, or does he show a lack of enthusiasm in your presentation? If the latter is the case, alter your teaching style to fit the style of the patient. Determine if the patient is bored. Do not maintain an agenda, just because it is yours. If the patient is not understanding the material, you need to shift directions. Watch the patient's eyes for clues as to whether he is a visual, auditory, or tactile learner. For example, visual learners prefer written literature that they can take home, study, and call with questions at a later time. Tactile (kinesthetic) learners may prefer to take a model hearing aid or ear and readily explore it. Auditory learners may simply sit and listen and then ask questions.

Determining a Patient's Level of Sophistication

Patients lie on a continuum in terms of the sophistication with which they process information. It can be difficult at times to determine if a patient comprehends crucial information. Because many patients are technically oriented, it is important to not talk down to them. Although some patients are in awe of an educated, experienced professional, credentials and authority do not particularly impress others.

- **Determine the patient's knowledge level through discussion.** Does the patient use technical terminology, and if so, does he use it appropriately? From one visit to the next, does the person retain previous information discussed? Does he build on previous conversations or literature that has been sent home?
- **Assess the comprehension.** Does the patient exhibit an understanding of facts? Is he able to summarize information or give appropriate examples of relevant information being discussed? Does the patient recognize unstated facts or infer from previous conversations? Does he analyze the explanation and ask relevant questions?
- **Is the person able to organize his thoughts?** Can the patient summarize and support his problems or concerns?

EXPLAINING RELEVANT ISSUES

Having determined the preferred way of instructing the patient, it is time to begin the formal education. As professionals gain experience, most will develop personal strategies for explaining information to patients in the office and will generate written material that can be sent home with them. Discussions and handouts can be supplemented with visual and hands-on demonstrations provided in the office as well as loaner videos and books (when desired). In the following section, aspects relevant to the process of hearing and the use of wearable amplification are described. *The information contained in the boxes, while quite basic for the audiologist, represents sample explanations to issues and frequently asked questions that can be given to the "average" patient.* Of course, the terminology may need to be altered (up or down) depending on the sophistication level of the individual. For example, technically knowledgeable patients may enjoy receiving a detailed handout or explanation of why hearing loss is much more complex than a simple loss of sensitivity. An example of this type of presentation may be found in Appendix 8–J in Chapter 8. Much of the following information can be easily adapted for use as handouts or even as website literature.

Anatomy and Physiology

A brief explanation of the function of the auditory system may help patients understand why hearing aids work well for some people and not others no matter how sophisticated the technology may be. The following sample explanation can be used with patients and/or adapted into a handout. An anatomy chart should be available to supplement this narration.

The ear is divided into three parts: the outer ear, the middle ear, and the inner ear. The outer ear includes the visible portion of the ear called the pinna or auricle and the ear canal. The pinna helps collect high-frequency sounds and direct them into the ear canal. The ear canal is a slightly curved cavity about 1 inch in length. It is lined with skin and glands that produce earwax, a sticky substance that lubricates the ear and helps prevent foreign objects from entering the ear. Normally, the ear canal has a "self-cleaning" mechanism, and the earwax flakes out of the ear by itself. Sometimes, however, too much earwax accumulates and an audiologist or physician may have to remove it. Usually, it is **not** advisable to use a Q-tip to try to remove it yourself, as you may push it in further or even injure your ear canal and/or eardrum. Sounds entering the ear canal vibrate the eardrum. The middle ear is located behind the eardrum. It is an air-filled space containing three tiny bones, commonly called the hammer, anvil, and stirrup (malleus, incus, and stapes). The outer and middle ear collectively make up the conductive system and are responsible for conducting sound energy to the inner ear. When the middle ear bones vibrate, the third bone (the stapes, or stirrup) pivots into and out of a "window" in the inner ear. This motion produces a wave of movement through the part of the inner ear called the cochlea. The cochlea is a snail-shaped bony structure housing thousands of tiny nerves called hair cells (because they look like hairs under a microscope) that sit along the entire length of the cochlea.

This wave stimulates the hair cells. High-pitched sounds cause a wave that stimulates the hair cells at the base of the cochlea (nearest to the middle ear), whereas low-pitched sounds travel the length of the cochlea resulting in activation of the nerve cells near the other end. Like a tiny keyboard, each place along the cochlea is sensitive or responsible for a particular sound.

The hair cells are connected to nerve fibers that go into the brain. When the nerve cells leave the cochlea and begin to enter the brain they come together to form the auditory nerve. Then the auditory nerve branches into portions of the brain ending in the auditory cortex. Thus, although we receive sounds in our ear, we actually hear in our brain.

In general, the human ear is capable of detecting sounds as soft as 0 dB (a soft whisper or leaves rustling) to as loud as 140 dB (the loudness of a jet engine). The ear can also hear sounds having a wide range of pitch. The pitch or frequency range is 20 to 20,000 Hz or vibrations per second. Low-pitched sounds might include a bullfrog, the pitch of a man's voice, and most vowel sounds. High-pitched sounds include a bird chirping, frying of an egg, and most consonant sounds.

Types of Hearing Impairments

Understanding the nature of one's hearing loss and how that disorder will be affected by amplification is important to convey.

Hearing loss may be caused by many different factors, including disease, infection, certain types of medication, exposure to loud noises, aging, and hereditary factors. The damage can occur at any point in the auditory system and is categorized according to site of damage or dysfunction: conductive, sensorineural, central, and mixed losses.

Continued

Conductive hearing loss is caused by a problem in the outer or middle ear. Examples include wax blockage in the ear canal, a hole in the eardrum, fluid in the middle ear, and a bony growth preventing movement of the middle ear bones. A conductive hearing loss decreases a person's ability to hear soft and sometimes moderately loud sounds. To hear better, a person with a conductive loss must turn up the volume or move closer to the sound source. Fortunately, this type of listener can usually understand words or hear sounds clearly when they are made louder. Because conductive hearing losses are usually caused by medical-related problems, they can often be treated with medication or surgery. Therefore, conductive hearing losses are not necessarily permanent.

Sensorineural hearing loss is caused by damage to or a disorder within the inner ear or on the auditory nerve. Viral infections, certain medications, aging, and noise exposure are common causes of sensorineural hearing loss. Beyond a loss of sensitivity, there are other distortions including loss of clarity in quiet and/or background noise. Sometimes, there is also difficulty tolerating loud sounds. Often, certain sounds are easier to hear than others. If a person has a high-frequency hearing loss, for example, he may be able to hear the louder, low-frequency sounds like the vowels "ah" or "au," but may not be able to hear the high-frequency, softer sounds of speech like the consonants "f" or "s." Because low-frequency sounds (the vowels) carry most of the loudness of speech, but high-frequency sounds (the consonants) are most important for understanding speech (clarity), individuals with high-frequency sensorineural hearing losses often remark that they can hear, but cannot understand.

Central hearing loss can occur from aging, brain injury, or other neurologic disorders producing difficulty in processing sound in the brain. This type of problem may result in loss of auditory memory, comprehension, or ability to complete other complicated listening tasks.

Hearing loss can be manifested in many ways. Depending on the nature of the loss, a listener might note a loss of sensitivity (ability to hear very soft sounds), a loss of clarity (ability to understand speech in quiet and/or in noise), difficulty tolerating loud sounds, or a combination of these.

Loss of Sensitivity

The hearing test measures the amount of loss of sensitivity. The degree of hearing loss may vary at different test frequencies and is shown on an audiogram (a chart showing how loud different pitch [frequency] sounds must be made to just be able to be heard by the listener). The loudness (intensity) is measured in dB HL (decibels on the Hearing Level scale). Degree of loss of sensitivity is usually classified as follows:

0 to 15 dB HL Normal hearing sensitivity

16 to 25 dB HL Slight Loss

26 to 40 dB HL Mild Loss

41 to 55 dB HL Moderate Loss

56 to 70 dB HL Moderately-Severe Loss

71 to 90 dB HL Severe Loss

91+ dB HL Profound Loss

Loss of Clarity

Loss of Clarity in Quiet.   Some hearing problems go beyond a simple loss of sensitivity. Often, a person has difficulty understanding words. This loss of clarity may be due to problems related to the cochlea or may be from the auditory nerve or the auditory system within the brain. It may result in impairment of a person's ability to understand speech clearly, even when it is sufficiently loud. A loss of clarity can be difficult to recognize because a person may not exhibit the typical signs of hearing loss such as requesting that voices or the television be turned up louder. Often, a person with this type of problem will accuse others of having poor diction or of mumbling. Sometimes individuals who have a loss of clarity appear to have a memory loss, a lack of concentration or disinterest. If the ability to understand words in quiet is severely impaired, even the best hearing aids may not be able to restore this function.

Continued

Loss of Clarity in Noise. Some sensorineural impaired listeners can understand quite well when speech is presented in a quiet environment. However, when listening in competing noise, they may experience a great deal of difficulty. To hear in background noise, these listeners may need the speech signal to be made much louder than the noise. Unfortunately, we often cannot control our environment so that these conditions occur. Older hearing aids were often unable to provide significant help in these situations. However, newer designed hearing aids and assistive listening devices are attempting to overcome these difficulties, with varying degrees of success.

Loudness Tolerance Problems

Abnormal loudness growth, technically called recruitment, is a problem that is experienced by most listeners with sensorineural impairments. Soft sounds have to be made louder to just be detected, but once they are loud enough to hear, just a slight increase might be interpreted as being quite loud, even intolerable. In reality, both listeners with sensorineural impairments and listeners with normal hearing define a sound as being uncomfortable or even intolerable at about the same level (usually 100 dB on the audiogram). The difference, however, is that the normal listener can detect a very soft sound (about 0 dB on the audiogram). Thus the *range* of usable sounds for the normal ear is about 100 dB (100 minus 0). But for the impaired ear, that range is much smaller, for example the threshold (the softest sound the particular impaired ear can detect) might be 60 dB, so if the loudest tolerable level is 100 dB, the range is only 40 dB. Therefore, all the sounds we encounter have to be crammed into a 40 dB range for the impaired ear, instead of a 100 dB range for the normal ear. This gives the impression of loudness growing very rapidly. This is an important factor in comfortably fitting hearing aids.

Hearing Aids

Hearing Aid Style

Patients should be informed of all options and then advised as to what is preferable for them.

Pictures or nonworking models showing the various styles of hearing aids should be available for demonstration to patients.

Behind-the-Ear (BTE) Hearing Aids. The BTE consists of a slender curved case that houses the electronic components. The instrument fits snugly over and behind the ear and connects to a short plastic tube that conducts the sound from the hearing aid to the plastic ear piece (called an earmold) that fits inside the ear.

Advantages
- Suitable for any age or degree of hearing loss
- Some consider them to be cosmetically appealing because of placement behind the ear
- Larger batteries and controls may be easier to manipulate than some smaller devices
- Less susceptible to ear wax problems
- Often has an on-off switch separate from the volume control
- Typically has superior telecoils
- May contain Direct Audio Input
- May contain directional and/or multiple microphones

Disadvantages
- Earmold and tubing need to be replaced periodically to maintain a good fit
- Outer ear must be somewhat intact to provide a place to sit on the ear
- Microphone placement is at the top and front of ear, so it does not mimic the real ear location
- Due to placement behind the ear, some consider them to be less cosmetically appealing

In-the-Ear (ITE) Hearing Aids. The ITE is typically available in a "full-shell" and "low profile" style. The hearing aid fits entirely into the ear in a custom-molded plastic case. The full-shell style fills up the entire bowl of the ear (called the concha). The low profile style, although also filling up the entire concha, is shallower and more recessed and is often cosmetically more attractive.

Advantages
- All-in-the-ear one-piece design is often considered cosmetically appealing

Continued

- Microphone placement more closely approaches natural hearing location
- May be easier to insert and remove for some individuals because it is all one piece
- May accommodate directional and/or multiple microphones
- May accommodate a telecoil

Disadvantages
- Increased chance for feedback due to closer proximity of microphone and receiver of hearing aid
- Battery door and volume control may be smaller, and thus more difficult to manipulate for some patients
- More susceptible to wax and moisture problems
- May require a pre-amp for the telecoil

In-the-Canal (ITC) Hearing Aids. The half-shell and ITC instruments are similar to the ITE hearing aids except they are smaller and more compact. The half-shell instrument, as its name implies, fills about half of the bowl of the ear. The ITC is less visible and primarily fills the ear canal with only the face of the hearing aid visible. Both of these instruments share many of the features of ITEs.

Advantages
- Enhanced cosmetic appeal
- Microphone placement more closely matches natural hearing
- May be easier to insert and remove for some individuals because it is all one piece

Disadvantages
- Increased chance of feedback due to the close proximity of the microphone and receiver
- Susceptible to earwax and moisture problems
- Controls and batteries are small and may be difficult for some individuals to manipulate
- Fewer options for venting due to smaller size
- May not have sufficient space for a telecoil
- Cannot presently accommodate directional or multiple microphones

Completely-in-the-Canal (CIC) Hearing Aids. These "nearly invisible" hearing aids are the smallest amplification devices available. They are typically made of hard plastic but sometimes have a soft, flexible shell material deep in the canal. Most do not have a volume control. The entire hearing aid sits within the ear canal, sometimes quite deeply.

Advantages
- The most cosmetically appealing
- May result in improved high-frequency amplification because of deeper position in the ear canal
- Microphone placement mimics natural hearing
- Takes advantage of directional cues supplied by the pinna and concha
- May be less affected by wind noise
- Improved telephone and headphone use with hearing aids
- If seated sufficiently deep in ear, may reduce occlusion effect

Disadvantages
- May not be appropriate for certain ear canals or when certain medical conditions exist
- Batteries are very small and may be difficult for some individuals to manipulate
- Almost no options for venting due to small size
- Increased chance of feedback because of the extremely close proximity of the microphone and receiver
- May be uncomfortable because of deep placement in the ear canal
- No available space for telecoil
- Typically more expensive than other styles

Linear Versus Compression Amplification

Hearing aids must have a means of controlling the maximum intensity reaching the listener's ear. An explanation of the options is important because it often defuses previous notions the patient may have based on the negative experiences of users of older hearing aids.

One of the major limitations of older hearing aids was that even though they were able to make soft sounds loud enough to hear, they also made loud sounds too loud. This created a situation where hearing aid users either constantly needed to adjust the volume control or rejected the hearing aids completely because sounds became uncomfortably loud for them. The type of cir-
Continued

cuitry that created this limitation in hearing aids was called linear, meaning that an equal amount of amplification was applied to sounds entering the hearing aid regardless of the loudness of the incoming sound. In other words, if a linear device provided 25 dB of amplification (or gain), a soft incoming sound of 20 dB would be increased to 45 dB and a loud incoming sound of 80 dB would be increased to 105 dB. The result of this type of amplification is that some soft sounds may not be audible and some loud sounds may be uncomfortable. Furthermore, many of the loud sounds pushed the hearing aid beyond its built-in limitations, thus creating a distorted, muffled signal.

As a result of these shortcomings, manufacturers and engineers designed nonlinear hearing aids. This circuitry, called compression, provides more gain for soft incoming sounds than it does for loud incoming sounds. Not only does this produce greater loudness comfort, but it results in less distortion for loud incoming speech sounds.

Single or Multiple Band Compression. Compression can be applied to hearing aids in either a single channel or multiple channels. Single channel means that when an incoming acoustic signal reaches a certain predetermined intensity (or loudness) level, the amount of amplification is reduced across the frequency range. It is almost like having an invisible finger adjusting the volume control. Unfortunately, although this will help maintain loudness comfort, certain high-frequency sounds could be reduced so much that they become inaudible.

Because most listeners' hearing sensitivity and loudness tolerance vary across the frequency range, compression can also be applied in multiple frequency channels. So, if a patient's hearing sensitivity and loudness tolerance is normal at one frequency but reduced at another frequency, the compression can be tailored to his needs. This also means that if a loud low-frequency sound enters the hearing aid, the amplification could be reduced only for the low frequencies without simultaneously reducing the volume of the high frequencies. This can play a role in lowering the perception of noise without adversely affecting the ability to understand speech.

Signal Processing

In the modern world of computers, patients have a right to be educated regarding options in technological advances.

Analog Hearing Aids

Analog processing has been the primary signal processing strategy used in hearing aids. Analog signals act like representations of the original sound wave in that they continually vary over time. Because sound waves are a physical event (as opposed to an electrical phenomenon), the wavelike motion of sound must be converted by the hearing aid microphone into an electrical signal that can be processed by the hearing aid. The electrical representation of the sound wave is "analogous" to the sound input. A commonly cited example of analog circuitry is an old phonograph. As the needle bumps its way over the notches and grooves in the record, the signal is transformed into analogous or similar electrical impulses that are passed through a speaker which, in turn, changes these analogous vibrations back into sound. Although technological advances for analog circuitry offer a wide variety of controls to manipulate sound output, they do not offer the manipulative ability of a digital circuit.

Digitally Programmable-Hybrid Hearing Aids

When an analog hearing aid uses digital control to adjust certain aspects of the amplification, the term digitally programmable is applied. This means that sound waves will be altered to an electronic signal by the microphone using an analog processing system. However, any adjustments made to the hearing aid with respect to amplification (gain), frequency response, and compression are done through digital control. In a conventional analog hearing aid, the flexibility and number of options are limited by space. Because digitally programmable hearing aids are interfaced with a computer during programming, space is not a concern. Additionally, the settings can be changed and saved in the hearing aid in one or more programs. Not all listeners who are hearing impaired require the use of programmable hearing aids. Furthermore, programmability, per se, does not imply superior listening performance.

The *advantages* of digitally programmable hearing aids are:
1. **Flexibility.** Changes in hearing can easily be accommodated, as can unusual audiometric configurations and fluctuating hearing loss.

Continued

2. **Multiple Programs.** It is often useful to be able to change the hearing aid characteristics (gain, frequency response, compression, etc.) depending on the environment one encounters. Multiple memory programmable hearing aids may have as few as two and as many as eight memories (or programs) that you can choose with the touch of a button in order to change program memories.

3. **Advanced Compression Circuitry.** Certain programmable hearing aids allow for advanced capabilities such as full dynamic range compression and multiple channel compression that are not available in analog systems.

The *disadvantages* of programmable aids are:
1. They are more expensive than conventional systems.
2. Not all audiologists in different parts of the country have access to the equipment (or knowledge) needed to work with them.
3. Programming requires more time by both the patient and the dispenser.

Digital Hearing Aids

Advancements in the ability to manufacture hearing aids that process sound digitally offer the potential for dramatic improvements over previously available instruments. Hearing aid researchers have been investigating the use of true digital technology for over a decade. They were held back because the increased power consumption needed to operate such instruments required the instruments to either be very large, or to be connected to a separate power source worn on the body. As a compromise, digitally programmable hearing aids were introduced on the market in the early 1990s. These devices represented an improvement over previous technology in that they were extremely flexible, could be fine-tuned, and had advanced compression capabilities. They were still somewhat limited, however, because although the hearing aids could be programmed by a computer (the digital portion), they still operated in an analog fashion. This meant that sound entering the hearing aid microphone would be amplified and filtered by a variety of electronic components. Because hearing is such a complex sense, the extent of filtering and amplifying required to correct an impairment added to the limitations of the hearing instrument by producing distortion and noise.

Digitization means that incoming sounds are converted to numbers, that are then analyzed and manipulated via a set of rules (algorithms) programmed into the chip controlling the hearing aid. The resultant digitized numbers are then manipulated according to the algorithm instructions, reconverted to an analog form (sound waves), and delivered to the ears, often producing cleaner signals than were commonly associated with analog technology hearing aids.

Digitization allows hearing aids to enact more advanced signal processing strategies than can be achieved in analog circuitry of the same size and power consumption. For example, some digital hearing aids divide the incoming sound into various bands (e.g., low frequency, mid frequency, and high frequency) and then selectively reduce the amount of amplification in specific bands depending on whether the hearing aid determines the main energy within that band to be predominantly speech or predominantly noise.

Hearing Aid Options

The specific needs of patients dictate which options they require and ultimately which specific models are recommended. Methods of determining patients' needs are described in Chapter 5.

Single Versus Multiple Programs

A hearing aid program refers to a specific set of parameters that optimize hearing in one or more listening environments. Single program hearing aids are set according to the user's most frequent listening needs. Single program hearing aids may be digitally programmable or even digital with immense opportunity for adjustments, but, outside of the volume, the hearing aid parameters cannot be changed after leaving the audiologist's office.

Some hearing aids have the ability to be switched from one program to another. This is beneficial if you have a lifestyle in which your listening environments differ dramatically throughout the day. Multiple programs are similar to having different hearing aids for various listening conditions or hearing needs.
Continued

Individuals with fluctuating loss benefit from the ability to switch programs as hearing changes. Others may benefit from this flexibility as well. For example, a mechanic may require a hearing aid that cuts out loud, low-frequency noise during the day. However, if later in the day he wishes to enjoy an opera performance, he might prefer a different hearing aid that enhances the quality of the sound across the vocal range of the performers. Short of having to buy and adjust to several hearing aids, multiple programs allow the hearing aid user to purchase one instrument and change that instrument's performance characteristics throughout the day by a switch located on the hearing aid or a remote control.

Multiple programs are not necessary or beneficial for everyone. Some individuals' lifestyles are such that their listening environments are similar throughout the day. When this is true, after a short time, people find themselves relying primarily on a single program. Because there is greater cost and fitting time involved, it would be unwise to buy this type of instrument and not make use of it. Also, some people find it difficult to manage more than one program. And, the programs must vary enough that the user can distinguish the differences and obtain benefit from them.

Remote Controls Versus Volume Controls Versus Automatic Adjustments

Some advanced compression hearing aids do not contain volume controls because the volume is automatically adjusted, depending on the loudness of the incoming sound. However, some experienced users of hearing aids having volume controls, seem quite hesitant to relinquish this feature. If you want to have a volume control, you have options including wheels and toggle switches on the instrument, or even remote controls. Of course, if you tend to lose things, a remote control may be risky and inappropriate.

Directional and Multiple Microphones

Most of the time, we face the person we are listening to. Noise, however, is often located in front of, behind, and/or to our sides.

Some hearing aids now contain directional or multiple microphones that "communicate" with each other in a manner such that sounds originating from the front of the hearing aid receive maximum amplification and sounds originating from the sides or behind the listener receive considerably less amplification. This effectively minimizes some of the annoying background noise that creates so much difficulty for listeners who are hearing impaired. The technology using these types of microphone arrays is very promising. This technology can be found in several different hearing aids but generally is limited to behind-the-ear or full shell in-the-ear hearing aids because of size restrictions.

Candidacy Issues

In the past several years hearing aid technology has progressed to the point where the issue of candidacy is based on your communicative needs rather than on your degree of hearing loss. The critical variable is whether you are having difficulty hearing or are experiencing increased stress and strain in your daily function. Amplification may simply relieve the strain of hearing, as opposed to making sounds louder or improving your score on a hearing test in which the percentage of words you can correctly identify is measured. However, this alone can be a very significant benefit. Ask yourself whether you are stressed or fatigued after a day of straining to listen. Ask yourself whether the ability to hear, but not understand, is adequate for your needs. Unselfishly examine whether you are becoming a burden to others because of breakdowns in communication. Remember that wearing a hearing aid is not necessarily a mark of infirmity, rather it is a mark of courtesy to others.

Monaural Versus Binaural Considerations

There are four primary reasons why binaural (two eared) listening is superior to monaural listening. They are:
1. **Better Hearing in Noise.** Numerous studies show that an individual's hearing in noise can be improved if the signal
Continued

reaching each ear is slightly different. We call this difference the phase of the sound. When the brain receives different signals at the two ears, it has the ability to compare the information and process the primary signal (usually speech) better than if the signal is received monaurally (one ear).

2. **Enhanced Signal Versus Noise by Optimizing Position.** Sound decreases in strength, mostly for high frequencies (those most responsible for consonant sounds), when it travels across the head. The amount it loses can be large enough that when added to the effects of a high-frequency hearing loss, the sound can not be heard if you are facing away from the person speaking to you.

3. **Improved Localization Ability.** We determine the location of sound by means of (a) interaural (between ear) differences in intensity, (b) interaural differences in relative time of arrival, and (c) interaural differences in spectral (pitch or frequency) cues. If sound is heard only in one ear, the brain cannot make use of these comparisons so it becomes more difficult to determine from where the sound is coming.

4. **Possible Deterioration of the Unaided Ear.** We hear in our brain, not in our ears. The ultimate goal of hearing aid fitting is not simply amplifying sound. It is also essential to retrain the brain (central auditory system). The old saying, "use it or lose it" is appropriate. Although the exact mechanism is still uncertain, there is scientific evidence that shows that clarity deteriorates at a faster pace in an ear that is unaided than it does in two ears that are both aided.

Adaptation Time

Depending on the individual, hearing aids may allow persons to experience sounds they have not heard before, if ever. Relearning takes place in the central auditory nervous system, not in the ear itself. Recent research findings suggest that listeners' understanding of speech may continue to increase when wearing a new amplification system for several months. This process is termed acclimatization. Most dispensing audiologists currently allow for a 1-month trial period with new hearing aids. If market conditions allow, trial periods may be extended to accommodate this acclimatization further. Above all, be patient and allow for acclimatization. The brain requires time to adjust to new sound, just as it requires time to get used to new eyeglasses.

Life Expectancy of Hearing Aids

Generally speaking, hearing aids should last for at least 5 years, or for as long as benefit continues if the hearing aids are properly maintained. The need for new hearing aids may occur if a patient's hearing status changes, but with the availability of programmable and digital hearing aids, changes can be made in the audiologist's office and should reduce the need to order new hearing aids merely because of changes in hearing status.

Assistive Listening Devices

One major goal of hearing devices is to enhance the relationship between the perceived loudness of the signal and the perceived loudness of the noise. Unfortunately, despite all the new technological advances, a basic problem remains for which wearable amplification falls woefully short. That problem relates to the physical distance between the microphone of the hearing aid and the source of the sound desired to be heard. Intensity decreases as physical distance increases. Unfortunately, most background noise surrounds the listener, so while the intensity of the speech decreases with distance, the intensity of the noise may not. This is one reason why hearing aids transmit sound so well if the speaker talks right into the microphone, but at longer, more realistic, distances, reception diminishes. It would be ideal to have the sound produced at the source transferred directly to your ear without losing any intensity. It is obviously impractical, however, to ask the speaker to move closer to your ear. One way of achieving this effect is with direct audio input, in which the speaker holds a microphone that is wired to the hearing aid itself near his or her mouth. Many hearing aid wearers are reluctant to ask the speaker to do this, however. An alternative approach is available through

Continued

infrared transmission, FM transmission, or inductance loop transmission. These systems are currently used in many theaters, concert halls, houses of worship, and households. One of the best uses is for television listening. The portable transmitter, usually a box smaller than most cable boxes, and microphone are located near the TV loudspeaker. The sound picked up by the microphone is then transmitted to a receiver, worn by the listener without any decrease in intensity. These devices can transmit with minimal distortion over a considerable distance (up to 50 feet). Assistive Listening Devices (ALDs) are becoming increasingly apparent in public places due to the recent legislative enactment of the Americans with Disabilities Act. Other, nonwearable devices that assist listeners who are hearing impaired include telephone amplifiers, vibrating alarm clocks, TV closed-caption decoders, inexpensive personal hand-held or body-worn amplifiers, visual alarm systems, and TDDs (telephone devices for the deaf).

Limitations of Hearing Aids

Perhaps the most common complaints expressed by patients relate to difficulties with loudness, the quality of amplified sound, and difficulty hearing in background noise. Directly addressing these issues can minimize subsequent disappointment by helping to establish realistic expectations.

Loudness

When addressing the issue of excessive loudness, it is essential to determine which sounds, and under what circumstances, seem too loud. If you think that most sounds are too loud, the hearing aid volume control or internal settings may need adjusting. If only some sounds are too loud, we need to consider the circumstances. For example, we may need to adjust the amplification for only certain pitches.

The impaired ear may negatively affect a person's ability to tolerate loud sounds. Soft sounds are not audible, yet when sounds are made a little louder, they seem disproportionately loud. Compression circuitry is designed to correct this situation, but the settings may need adjustments and fine-tuning.

Also, when patients get new hearing aids, they sometimes do not realize how different the world will sound. It is possible that you may be experiencing the normal fluctuation of sounds. It may help to ask others if they too find the particular environment to be too loud for them.

The bottom line, however, is that it is not acceptable for hearing aids to sound too loud. If they do, they need to be adjusted. Modern hearing aids should prevent most sounds from becoming uncomfortably loud. So if this is occurring, do not hesitate to schedule an appointment for an adjustment.

Sounds Are Not Natural

There are many reasons why hearing aids do not sound perfectly natural. Of course, some are related to the fact that the hearing aids contain loudspeakers that are very tiny and are powered by a small battery. Thus, sound is not reproduced with complete accuracy. Another reason is related to your hearing loss rather than the hearing aids. This complaint can be difficult to solve until we determine what your expectation is for "natural" hearing. Often, hearing loss is in the high-frequency range. Because hearing tends to decrease gradually, sounds that seem natural or normal for you may not represent the entire pitch range. In other words, it may be "natural" for you to hear mostly the low-frequency part of each word. For example, if I say the word "stop" you may be used to hearing mostly the "o" and detecting the other sounds mostly from context, lipreading, and other cues. Therefore, it is possible that when hearing aids restore those high-frequency sounds, it does indeed sound different or unnatural to you. Thus, it is important to practice listening with your hearing aids so that you can become accustomed to amplified sound.

Background Noise

Our world is a noisy place. Every day our ears are inundated with sounds. Some are pleasant, meaningful sounds such as the
Continued

voices of our loved ones. Other sounds, such as jet planes flying overhead, are less important. For us to cope with all the sounds in our environment, we learn to ignore many of the day-to-day background noises and tune in to the important sounds. Nevertheless, we still "hear" those sounds. If you went to bed with normal hearing and awoke the next morning with a significant hearing loss, you would notice and miss all of those sounds. In fact, they can actually help us stay connected to our environment.

When you lose your hearing gradually, however, sounds such as wind noise, clocks ticking, crickets chirping, clothing noise, footsteps, water running, and motor noises fade into the background and become less noticeable until they are completely inaudible. Therefore, you can easily forget what sounds should be there. In some ways, this is pleasing to people because they become accustomed to a peaceful and quiet world. However, the ability to listen selectively to important sounds and tune out noise may also diminish. Because these sounds aren't terribly interesting to most people, the brain suppresses them. But when the sounds are amplified and suddenly "reappear" to the person who is hearing impaired, the brain will tend to focus on them.

Some hearing aids are better than others at minimizing the effects of background noise. For example, as mentioned earlier, some digital hearing aids attempt to reduce the annoyance of noise by lowering amplification only for those bands where noise is the predominant signal. However, because noise is comprised of many of the same frequencies as speech, it is virtually impossible to "shut out" noise without also adversely affecting the quality of the speech signal. In reality, shutting out all background noise would take the "color" away from the world. It would be like living in a visual world of all black and white.

Occasionally, there are individuals who cannot get used to listening in background noise, despite a trial with even the most sophisticated amplification. That does not mean that these individuals must suffer a lifelong exposure to noise and discomfort. There are other means of improving one's ability to listen in background noise. From a technological standpoint, there are assistive listening devices that can provide help. Also, many people can practice good listening and speech reading techniques that can assist them in gradually improving their listening skills over time.

Occlusion Effect

When you speak, the vibration from your voice box actually produces a vibration in your ear canal. Normally this low-frequency vibration escapes into the air when your ear is unblocked. However, if you block your ear with a hearing aid, an earmold, or even your finger (go ahead and try it), you will notice that your voice sounds as if it has shifted into the blocked ear. This happens because these low-frequency vibrations have had their escape route cut off. It may sound to you as if you are talking in a barrel or experiencing an echo. This "occlusion effect" is also responsible for some of the difficulty hearing aid users (and non hearing aid users) experience when chewing food (particularly crunchy foods like carrot sticks or potato chips). To some extent, you will automatically adapt to the occlusion effect in time. However, the effect can be minimized by:

1. keeping the ear as open as possible;
2. reducing low-frequency gain;
3. using an earmold or shell in your ear that is deep enough that it makes contact with the bony inner half of your ear canal; however, this may be uncomfortable because the skin is much thinner in that part of the canal.

Feedback

There are two types of acoustic feedback: that produced internally from the hearing aid, indicating an aid in need of repair, and the more common external feedback produced by a leakage of amplified sound out of the ear canal and back into the microphone of the hearing aid. Leakage can occur if the earmold or hearing aid shell does not fit well, if the device is not properly inserted, if your hand is placed near the microphone, or if the sound path is deflected inside of your ear by debris, earwax, or hair. Usually, external feedback can be corrected by:

1. reinserting, or possibly remaking the earmold (or in-the-ear shell);

Continued

2. plugging, or reducing the diameter of any vents in the hearing aid or earmold (coupling) system;
3. reducing the amount of high-frequency gain (typically an unacceptable trade-off because of the resultant loss of high-frequency audibility); or
4. altering the frequency peak of the hearing aid with acoustic dampers, filters, or electronic adjustments.

Recently, some manufacturers have introduced digital feedback reduction in which feedback is sensed by the hearing aid, the pitch of the feedback is analyzed, and a new signal having the opposite phase relationship is generated, thus canceling out the feedback. It is important that you realize that feedback should not be acceptable to you or others around you. Remind your family and friends to alert you when the feedback occurs so that you can make it stop.

Battery Life

There are times when an unusually short battery life can signal a problem with the hearing aid. For example, if you typically get 12 to 14 days from a battery and suddenly batteries are lasting only 3 days, both the hearing aid and your ear should be examined. This problem may be caused by bad batteries, improper battery drainage or other electronic/circuitry problems with the instrument, or wax blockage in the ear or in the hearing aid receiver that forces the hearing aid to work much harder to amplify the sound. When this occurs, you may be turning the hearing aid up much higher than usual without realizing it, thus increasing the drainage of the battery.

Hearing Aid Repairs

Hearing aids are exposed to many elements in and out of the ear. The hearing aid's worst enemies are earwax and moisture because they cause damage to the delicate parts. Even when they are meticulously cleaned and cared for outside of the ear, perspiration and earwax can create havoc to the electronics. While manufac-turers work to isolate and strengthen the electronics from these kinds of elements, we ask them to make them smaller and smaller to keep up with our desire for a cosmetically appealing instru-ment. We would never expect our other electronic devices to con-tinue to work all day long, day after day, under these circumstances. Subsequently, we must understand why hearing aids may appear to break down often. Remember that even a slight amount of earwax blocking the sound opening of the hear-ing aid can significantly reduce the amplified sound. With that in mind, there are things we can do to minimize the problems. Au-diologists can suggest several techniques and products that might prove beneficial.

Importance of Visual Aids

Most of us do not realize how much we rely on speechreading. We learn speechreading at an early age and develop the skill nat-urally, even if we do not have hearing loss. Let me show you how much it helps. First, let's have a short face-to-face conversation. Now, I will keep my voice at the same level. However, I am going to cover my face with a "listening hoop" that will eliminate visual cues without affecting the sound. Do you think visual cues make a big difference?

When we have the advantage of seeing a person speaking, we pick up lots of important cues. Many sounds produced on the lips can be determined with little or no hearing by a skilled speechreader. There are also changes in facial features, gestures, and body language that can supplement our listening to provide us with a better understanding of spoken language. For example, if someone says "I saw a rat in my garage," but all you heard was "I saw a —at in my garage," there would be important cues in lip reading and expression that might help you figure out what was said. If the speaker had said cat instead of rat, he probably would not show disgust or fear on his face and, if he liked cats, his ex-pression may be of excitement or happiness. That is why you can understand better when looking at the speaker. This is a good practice and should be fostered whenever possible.

Specific Office Policies

Cost Issues

The reason hearing aids cost so much are:

1. They are sold in relatively low volume as compared to other electronic devices such as stereos.
2. The amount of time and money spent by manufacturers on research and development is considerable. One manufacturer claims to have spent over $20 million developing a single model.
3. The amount of time spent by the audiologist with a patient is very significant. An average of 5 direct contact hours is spent during the first year a patient receives hearing aids. This time is critical for new users, particularly to assist the adjustment process.

Mail Order

Some patients ask if it would be better (translation: cheaper) to purchase their hearing aids by mail order or through the Internet.

Products offered through the mail or via the Internet advertise lower prices because these suppliers do not need to provide you with any of the fitting and counseling services that are critical for the proper fitting and use of a hearing aid. Hearing losses and hearing needs are unique and require customization of the product and services to ensure the greatest benefit. The one size fits all philosophy of these mail order suppliers cannot provide you with the best possible hearing. This view is strongly supported by the FDA and most state legislatures.

Insurance and Medicare

Medicare will not pay for hearing aids because the federal government has specifically excluded hearing aid purchases from Medicare coverage. Efforts have been made to have them covered, but the federal government's objective at this time is to control or reduce the cost of Medicare coverage overall. They are very reluctant to add new services or products to the list. Simply put, many politicians have said it would bankrupt the system because of the high number of subscribers in need of hearing aids.

Most insurance companies and the employers who provide insurance have not recognized the importance of hearing health coverage and view it as a benefit that would only serve a small portion of the employees. Subsequently, it is necessary to check with the insurance company on an individual basis to determine if your policy includes this type of coverage. If so, it is also necessary to determine at what level they will pay. Although some insurance companies will pay for hearing aids and services in full, most will pay only a portion, if at all.

Bargaining for Prices

Our prices reflect the quality of products and services we provide. Price cannot be viewed in a vacuum. We are not simply talking about the price of the product, but the value of the total package. You must be sure you are comparing apples to apples: the same size, the same technology, the same warranty, and the same follow-up care. Higher quality products and service by more experienced audiologists as well as extended warranties equate to higher cost. However, we believe that our patients have a high level of satisfaction and receive greater benefit from their hearing aid purchase over a longer period of time.

CONCLUSIONS

The importance of answering truthfully but matching the level of your answers to the level of sophistication of patients cannot be overstated. Providing patients with handouts and brochures discussing these, and other issues, is helpful and will be appreciated.

Once the patient has received a thorough and clear explanation of his hearing impairment and has accepted the need for hearing aids, the professional must now turn her attention to the difficult task of determining which style and model of hearing aids to recommend. In keeping with the spirit of this book, remember that the patient should play an active role in the decision-making process. To do so, however, he must be made aware of all the options available. In Chapter 5, Marlene Bevan describes the many options and features of modern hearing aids that must be considered and matched to the needs of a given patient (or "client", the term preferred by Bevan). Open communication obtained through good counseling is critical in determining these needs. The importance of acquainting patients with state-of-the-art technology cannot be overstated. Assumptions regarding a patient's willingness or financial ability to try premium hearing aids should not be made lightly. All patients deserve the opportunity to experience the best hearing possible.

5

Matching Technology to the Hearing Needs of the Client

■ Marlene Bevan, Ph.D. ■

Matching advanced technology to the needs of the client begins substantially before the clinician explains the hearing aid recommendation. It begins with the design of an interactive hearing health care system that provides the consumer with an opportunity to share information about the experience of being hearing impaired and to hear information about the options and solutions to hearing impairments. Before the process of matching technology can begin, the consumer must establish a relationship with the provider and, eventually, the entire hearing health care team. The entire team, the front office staff, the hearing aid technicians or fitters, and the clinical or audiology staff become part of the partnership to facilitate the best rehabilitative outcome. Each member contributes to the client's feeling of trust, the feeling of being cared about, and the feeling of support throughout a period of significant behavioral change as the client makes the decision to utilize amplification. The partnership begins with a coordinated marketing effort to educate the consumer who is hearing impaired.

Throughout this chapter, the terms "consumer," "customer," and "client" are used. These terms are not interchangeable. In the hearing health care field, a *consumer* is the individual seeking information and may or may not be the individual with a hearing impairment. The customer is the individual who seeks assistance from the hearing health care practice. He is not committed to follow your recommendations or to accept your advice. The *client* is the individual who ultimately responds to your counsel, accepts your advice, and follows your suggestions for technology. Clients are not patients seeking treatment for injury or disease. They have engaged your professional services and seek your professional counseling to guide them in the selection of the best amplification. The ability to transform consumers into clients is essential to the success of the hearing instrument fitting process.

THE SAFE SOURCE FOR HEARING TECHNOLOGY

The hearing health care practice must be positioned in the marketplace as a safe source of information about hearing loss and hearing aids. This can be achieved by marketing activities that educate the consumer without risk. Seminars, consumer articles, radio, and television appearances can be used to promote both your knowledge of the problems of the hearing impaired and your individual practice. Throughout these events, the importance of establishing a relationship with an audiologist should be stressed. The audiologist is the best source of information for each individual's unique communication needs. Hearing aids may not be the only answer to communication problems. By contacting an audiologist consumers will learn about their unique hearing problems and what options exist to improve their communication abilities. Each marketing activity should conclude with this fact. Marketing activities firmly establish an expectation of consumer safety and underscore the need for a hearing health care relationship based on trust. As soon as the consumer approaches the hearing health care professional, the rehabilitative partnership should be initiated. To do this most effectively, and to understand the importance of matching technology to the individual's needs, we must have a better understanding about the population we will serve.

UNDERSTANDING THE HEARING IMPAIRED MARKETPLACE

There are approximately 28 million prospective clients in the marketplace of the hearing impaired. The largest population currently served are those 65 years of age and older. However, this may change as the Baby Boomers approach their sixties and presbycusis becomes a significant factor in their lives. They will soon become aware that a developing hearing impairment will affect their quality of life, lifestyle satisfaction, and overall general health status. Baby Boomers represent a unique type of consumer and will require services and goods designed specifically to their demands. These consumers have distinctive buying characteristics and are not known to postpone consumer gratification, nor do they routinely choose an option that is less than the best. They have a history of demanding immediate attention, quality products and solutions, and ongoing service.

RECOMMENDATIONS FOR DISSATISFIED CONSUMERS

Despite the vast number of adults with hearing loss who might benefit from amplification, only about 6 million now utilize amplification. Of those, less than half report satisfaction with their devices. In a marketplace of incredible opportunity, we have failed to reach a significant number who could benefit from hearing aids, and a majority of those we have reached feel that the solutions they obtained neither meet their expectations nor solve their communication problems.

An examination of hearing aid sales by technology type suggests that we continue to offer the same types of solutions that have previously failed to satisfy consumers who are hearing impaired. Although there are more potential solutions, and more options than simple linear and nonlinear, nonprogrammable circuits, these continue to be the most popular recommendations in our field. These types of hearing aids score depressingly low in consumer satisfaction studies. In 1996, 86% of hearing instruments dispensed were nonprogrammable technology. Of those, 48% were nonprogrammable, nonlinear technology (Strom, 1998). Given the lack of success experienced by consumers who are hearing impaired with conventional hearing aids, it is puzzling that a majority of hearing professionals continues to recommend linear, nonprogrammable technology.

There are hearing instrument solutions available that provide higher consumer satisfaction, but these instruments are not regularly chosen by consumers or dispensers. This situation is presently changing, albeit slower than optimal. Digitally programmable technology, including hybrid programmable units, rose from 29% of the market in 1996 to 39% in 1997. Digital Signal Processing (DSP), promising the fitter the ability to provide enhanced sound quality, flexibility of fitting, and listening comfort in a variety of listening situations, is chosen by consumers and/or dispensers less than half of the time. DSP units, reportedly preferred by listeners who are hearing impaired in difficult listening situations (Kochkin, 1996), rose from a mere 6% in 1996 to just 12% of sales in 1997. It is difficult to understand the slow growth of sales for this type of advanced technology when consumer complaints of poor performance in difficult listening situations with conventional hearing aids are so high.

WHY ARE SOME PROFESSIONALS RELUCTANT TO RECOMMEND PREMIER HEARING AID TECHNOLOGY?

Perhaps, many hearing specialists fail to match the hearing needs of clients to the best hearing aid technology available because these professionals are afraid of the cost of the instruments. Programmable or digital signal processing hearing instruments can cost the consumer almost twice the amount of conventional hearing aids. Many specialists, lacking confidence in the technology they provide and lacking significant experience with consumerism on their own, have become economically fixated on the purchase price of high technology hearing aids. By fixating on price, they may ignore the potential benefits and fail to present those benefits to frustrated consumers, many of whom may be quite willing to pay more for premium hearing aids if they indeed help them to hear better.

Some hearing professionals have a fear of new technology and/or have not taken the time to learn about it. New technology requires more clinician education and perhaps may involve more professional time. Some professionals may worry whether new hearing technology will adequately meet the expectations of their clients. They may fret about whether they can program the instruments successfully and whether the devices perform well enough to justify their recommendation. The clinician's lack of knowledge and experience with newly released devices can contribute to a lack of enthusiasm for these products. If the clinician has difficulty understanding or explaining the mechanics of the system or finding the appropriate cables and attachments, then the hearing aid fitting appointment could become an embarrassing demonstration of professional shortcomings.

There may also be the fear of the loss of future hearing aid sales. If programmable units are provided, will the client return only for reprogramming visits? Will new hearing aid sales markedly decrease? Once the client relationship is established, audiologists delivering additional follow-up services can seize the opportunity to deliver audiologic rehabilitation, update the client on new technology, and market companion products that improve the use of hearing aids. If the client's interaction with the hearing practice continues to improve his communication performance and skills, then that client will continue to feel satisfied with his hearing aids and the communication solutions that have been provided. When your client is satisfied with his hearing aid experience he can become a valued referral source for the practice and will not hesitate to recommend you to his friends and family members with hearing loss. Thus, improving rehabilitation results can improve the viability of our practices.

Whatever the cause, dispensers need to overcome their fear of premier devices because these hearing aids provide greater user satisfaction (Kochkin, 1996). Therefore, it is the professional and ethical obligation of the clinician to maintain her continuing education and become adept at managing these modern, state-of-the-art products.

WHAT ARE CONSUMERS REALLY AFRAID OF?

Cost concern may rank higher for the hearing aid professional than for many consumers. With a history of 50 to 60 years of consumerism, the typical individual who is hearing impaired in all likelihood has a purchasing history including homes, vehicles, boats, properties, optional surgical procedures, appliances, and countless other electronic gadgets. *Fear of cost is not an unusual initial response to a large investment; however, it is the fear of the purchase without value that overwhelms most people. If the item purchased has no intrinsic value, then the individual has wasted the purchase price and the problem once thought solved with the purchase remains unaffected. The discussion of cost must take place in the context of value. When the hearing aid solution works to solve the problem of the consumer, then the investment will be justified.*

Consumers understand the complexity of technology. There is no reason to assume that adults who are hearing-impaired are naive consumers, or that they will be unable to identify with the professional's discomfort with technology. The technology we now use routinely may have at one time or another posed a significant challenge to most adults. Answering machines and VCR's required some degree of skill to program accurately. Many consumers may have given up on achieving the task. Programming difficulty with hearing aid technology is not an unforgivable offense and it is not unreasonable to request manufacturer support for unusual fitting circumstances encountered during fitting. Although this does not give license to unprepared hearing aid professionals, clients may understand these issues and will not automatically lose faith in the provider's fitting skills if the professional utilizes manufacturer support during unusual fitting circumstances.

Consumers have a right to hear discussions of the full spectrum of hearing aid technology. The marketplace today is full of confusing terms and marketing promises, and clinicians have a responsibility to present the full range of hearing options to clients. Avoidance of the thorough presentation of options is not good hearing health care. As a professional, you must inform clients of their options before you can expect them to make a decision or follow a recommendation regarding which options are best for their unique hearing problems. If you avoid this discussion, you may be caught later by clients who feel betrayed because they were never told about a particular option. If you work to gain the trust of clients, and then exclude them from the decision making process, then you have violated their trust. *When options are withheld from clients, the hearing professional becomes responsible for any of the perceived shortcomings of the solution.* But, before you have the opportunity to present the options to your clients, you must attract consumers, convince customers, and gain the confidence of clients who are hearing impaired.

THE INITIAL APPOINTMENT

The initial appointment marks the beginning of the relationship of trust with the customer. If you are successful, the customer will choose to become a valued client of the practice. He arrives at this appointment to investigate the possibility of purchasing goods or services from you. However, he is not committed to follow your counsel or accept your recommendations. You must develop a relationship before you attempt to diagnose or educate the customer. The process of matching technology to needs and hearing aid fitting is most effective when counseling is framed in the context of a relationship.

Begin the relationship by "downloading" the customer. You must find out what the customer understands about the hearing health care system and hearing aids. Pay attention. Attentiveness is the foundation of this relationship. This is not the time for familiarity, jocularity, or judgmental response. If the customer complains that frequent and repeated purchase of hearing aids have all yielded the same unhappy results, resist the urge to comment on the client's poor judgment of hearing aid professionals or his susceptibility to fraudulent advertisements. Sympathize with the experience. Acknowledge the client's disappointment in his failure to obtain successful hearing solutions. Encourage discussion of the customer's feelings. Don't deny his experiences. If all his friends are unhappy with hearing aids, and he fears that hearing loss is isolating him from his social activities, then that is a frightening dilemma for him. If you deny that while attempting to convince him of the efficacy of hearing aids you will fail to gain his confidence.

Take the time to talk about your own experience with hearing aids. Build the prospective client's confidence in your ability to provide successful strategies or options for hearing loss. Introduce your years of experience, the numbers of fittings you have accomplished, and your satisfaction in helping people with hearing loss overcome this potential handicap. You need not engage in a long-winded dissertation about yourself, but it is appropriate and necessary to inform the client about your competency. Once accomplished you should also explain the protocols in place within your practice that help all clients succeed in the search for their unique solution to hearing loss. These might include satisfaction guarantees, evaluation periods, and follow up services to assure continued success over time.

Don't assume that you understand the type of hearing help your client is seeking. It is tempting to classify aided benefit in terms of measured aided sound-field thresholds and real-ear target gain, but you may miss the client's unique definition of the reality of hearing improvement. Help clients define what success will sound like. The COSI, Client Oriented Scale of Improvement (discussed in Chapters 7 and 8), is an effective method of obtaining this information. Ask the question, "What would you like to hear better?" Or, "Where would you like to hear better?" and record the client's response. Solicit three or four specific situations in which clients are willing to define success by an improvement in their hearing. If you know what clients want to hear, then you must decide if successful amplification will provide it. For example, many clients will tell you that they are frustrated by the inability to hear their spouses' conversation. However, in further discussion, you may find that they are frustrated by the spouses' constant communication from the next room, while washing dishes, when they are involved in reading the paper. Improved hearing ability may help the client in these situations, but it is the poor communication practice that may be at the root of the problem. If clients think hearing aids will solve these problems, and then they do not, any other improvements may also be discounted because you have not improved the ability to "hear my spouse." Define the communication problem carefully so that amplification results in improved communication. For example, "I have difficulty hearing my spouse at mealtime. This is worse when we are at a restaurant, with another couple or with our children and grandchildren." Now agree on the situations that occur most frequently, and get the client to agree that in each situation, if communication were improved, it would be considered a success. During the fitting process you must refer to these situations to measure your success in the amplification process and to assure both you and your client that you are continuing to improve hearing performance as you have both agreed to it and defined it. Provide clients' "sound of success" and you provide the successful sound solution.

If customers believe that they will hear what they want to hear and feel that you and your practice are qualified to provide the service necessary to help them succeed, then get them to commit to finding the solution with you. State your intentions clearly. Ask your customers, "If amplification could improve your ability to understand your spouse at mealtime when your are at home, in restaurants, and with a small group of friends, would you be ready to use hearing aids?" If they agree to the use of hearing aids that provide specific improvements, these customers become clients of the practice. A hearing aid fitting within the framework of this client-centered relationship has a high probability of success.

Gathering Diagnostic Information

The diagnostic information we generate provides a scientific reference for many clients' observations about the communication handicap imposed by the hearing impairment. All clients generate a distinct set of observations, even when the loss measurements may be identical to several other clients you are counseling. Testing may be a standard routine for clinicians, but clients find themselves in a very stressful and strange experience. Many audiology evaluations simply last too long. Adults grow weary while straining to respond as soon as they hear the "just barely audible sounds" presented first in their good ear and then in their poorer ear. When adults have difficulty sorting out the first set of instructions, many clinicians have heard themselves utter the second set of instructions with a condescending tone. This experience can only become more upsetting to clients. Minimize the basic level of client anxiety during the evaluation by moving through diagnostics quickly and efficiently, without exhausting or frustrating them. Be encouraging and understanding about any discomfort the assessment may have caused. At the conclusion of testing, remember to thank clients for their cooperation. Reaffirm that the testing results yielded important information that help you to understand the basis of their communication problems and will help you both make the right choices for hearing solutions.

Share the results of your evaluation in simple terms. Report your findings in a positive, but direct manner (refer to Chapter 4 for a detailed discussion on conveying technical results in lay terminology).

Clinician: Mr. Smith, as a result of today's testing, I found that your hearing ability is about the same in each ear. You have a sensorineural hearing loss. This means that the hearing loss is permanent and hearing will not be restored by the use of medicines or surgery. More important, it means that in many situations, conversations can become garbled unless you pay close attention or there is only one speaker to whom you are listening. You mentioned to me earlier that when you attend meetings and several speakers participate, it might be difficult for you to stay involved in the conversation. I think that's a good example of the effect of this kind of hearing loss.

Don't feel compelled to explain degree of hearing loss and reduced speech recognition ability; instead, explain what sounds the client can hear and how clearly or easily he is able to recognize speech without visual cues. Whenever possible, use your test results to validate the client's observations about his hearing. Finally, explain why (or why not) he will be a good candidate for amplification.

Clinician: Mr. Smith, although there is no way to restore your normal hearing, you are an excellent candidate for the use of amplification. You've shared lots of examples of situations in which you would be pleased if better hearing was possible for you. You're an active individual and it seems that a large part of enjoying the quality of your lifestyle depends on hearing better in several key situations.

Emphasize courtesy and respect for your clients to underscore the working partnership you want to create. Review the specific communication situations to come up with enough information to help you as a clinician understand the situations in which amplification will be required to function efficiently. Use this process to strengthen the client-centered partnership and your eventual recommendations. Together, you have defined the client's hearing potential, and this information combined with the information about the impact of the hearing loss on the client's lifestyle is essential as you attempt to match technology to hearing needs.

INTRODUCING HEARING AID TECHNOLOGY
TO TODAY'S CONSUMER

The term "technology" is familiar to Baby Boomers, and many Boomers require little introduction to the concept. They access daily information about the latest in automotive, communications, and personal-electronic technology in newspapers, television, radio, and on the Internet. They are a culture of "technology-fans," ready to embrace the latest and the greatest innovations. In many cases they have already started their research to become well informed about the benefits and the shortcomings of the technology they desire before they seek professional help.

SELLING TECHNOLOGY TO THE INFORMED CONSUMER

The marketing of technology has a less than confidence inspiring history. New technology becomes obsolete as fast as we can purchase it. Once sold on the advantages of new technology, it is all too often not possible to "get there" from the old technology. Owners of last year's Computer Operating System or the Super-Nintendo before the Nintendo 64 may have found that they have no method to upgrade their purchases. The previous investment became obsolete and new technology was not necessarily compatible with the old technology. Previous investments were no longer useful and needed to be replaced in order to obtain the promised new benefits. You must constantly replace last year's purchase with next year's model. This creates a distrustful situation that accompanies the marketing of technology and it is not out of step with the distrust present in the hearing industry.

PRESENTING HEARING AID TECHNOLOGY TO CONSUMERS

Stories about consumer victims of the hearing health care field appear frequently in the media, and accusations of false advertising claims cloud the hearing industry today almost as loudly as they did more than 20 years ago. These stories have become the "folk lore" of the hearing health care system. The fragmentation of the professionals involved in the delivery of hearing health care and the confusing presentation of technical terminology make it all the more difficult to establish professional credibility. Each attempt by the government to legislate consumer safety brings yet another wave of consumer distrust. Ignoring the benefits of technology, however, will not settle trust issues in the mind of the consumer.

Perhaps because technology is difficult to present, clinicians fail to provide advanced technology options to all their clients. Without suggesting technology options, they may order hearing aids without specifying circuitry or fitting matrix. If these clinicians are not interested in performance differences, they abdicate professional responsibility in this vital aspect of the fitting process. Whatever the reason, a rational presentation of technology is frequently absent. All technology that relates to clients' specific communication issues must be presented in addition to the compromises associated with less advanced technology. *Good clinicians must advocate for their clients' best choices.*

THE UNPREDICTABLE AND HEARING AID TECHNOLOGY

Clients may frequently pose problems or situations that clinicians cannot predict. Personal adjustment problems, reliability in challenging environments of high humidity, or extreme dirt, and overall client satisfaction cannot be predicted with complete accuracy. A truthful discussion of the unknown is important and furthers the honesty in the process of forming a lasting relationship with your client.

The pace of new developments is an event that cannot be predicted. This poses a risk to consumers. If the technology purchased is a compromise (e.g., the best performance for the best style), and the clinician knows that there will shortly be a better style available with better performance, then there is an ethical obligation to discuss what is known. It is also important to express your professional opinion, but recognize that any decision to purchase now or to wait ultimately belongs to the client. In the computer industry, a leading manufacturer has begun to educate the market to accept lease option without purchase as insurance against obsolete technology. The consumer agrees to pay for the computer monthly and in a minimum of 2 years, can return the computer for a more advanced system at some additional cost and a continued monthly payment. This purchase program, called "your ware," is centered on removing the fear of purchasing technology that soon becomes obsolete. A comparable response might be beneficial for purchases within the hearing health care field if clinicians believe in the superiority of the technology and the likelihood of increasing speed in the developing advances.

HEARING NEEDS ARE QUALITY OF LIFE ISSUES

An investment in hearing technology is an investment in the return to quality of life. The development of the client-clinician partnership enables you to understand the quality of life issues faced by your clients. Certainly the communication needs for life quality expressed by the Baby Boomer and the nursing home resident are exceptionally different, but each should be informed of the range of options available. Clients' ultimate choices are highly related to the clinician's presentations. Therefore, you must understand the human issues before you can appropriately match technology to their needs.

CLIENTS WILL TELL YOU, IF YOU ARE READY TO LISTEN

Most clients know which issues are key to their successful use of hearing aids. If you ask them, they are usually willing to share this information. But you must be prepared to ask. *Recommending the appropriate circuitry depends on your understanding of the client's lifestyle issues.* The counseling process builds clients' confidence in your ability. At this point in the initial consultation, you have completed the initial hearing needs assessment and the diagnostic assessment, and you can now again ask about the client's understanding of hearing aids.

Set the tone with a friendly, open body position. This is accomplished by uncrossing your legs, unfolding your arms, and sitting forward, slightly. Folded arms or legs across your body communicate a "closed" nonverbal message. If you are unsure of the best initial position, mimic the body position of your client. If it feels "closed," establish eye contact during the interview and slowly move to a more "open" position. If you make small purposeful changes and then wait, clients will often mimic your change. Set the physical stage by sitting face to face with your clients, one-to-one, utilizing good eye contact. Encourage the client's use of eye contact by communicating your nonverbal feelings of empathy in this configuration. Send the signal that you are ready to listen and to pay attention. Good clinicians are good listeners. Phrase your questions in an open-ended manner that requires more than one-word answers. Encourage clients to elaborate by asking them to "tell me more about that." Often there are periods of silence during this process. (See Chapter 2 for further suggestions on this issue.) Clients may search for the words to share their feelings. The inexperienced clinician may feel uncomfortable and try to fill these silences with chatter. This is ultimately unproductive and diverts attention from your questions. Ask additional questions when you suspect that clients have completed the answer as best as they can. Again, ask questions to learn what they know about hearing aids. Ask what event motivated them to search for hearing help at this time. Most of our clients with age-related hearing loss know other friends or family members with hearing loss. Ask what they have observed about the behavior of friends or family members using hearing aids. Ask what they think of the experience of their friends or family members with hearing aids. Ask what experiences they would like to have if they decide to use hearing aids. Ask and then listen carefully. The information that clients offer can be used to determine the appropriate technology recommendations. Clients' observations are the clearest indications of what technology must do to succeed for them. If they will share their feelings, you will know what they most want hearing aids to do for them and what they are most concerned about that hearing aids will do to them.

SELECTING HEARING AID OPTIONS

The availability of the following options should be discussed with clients.

User Controlled Volume Settings

Your client may tell you about friends or family members who constantly adjust the volume control on their hearing aids. This may be viewed as a negative or positive behavior. The client will generally tell you which it is. If he does not, ask him directly. He may object to hearing aid devices that require frequent attention or adjustment. He may question the need to "fiddle" constantly with the settings on the hearing aids. He may request hearing instrumentation that is already set for him, or he may talk about the benefit of controlling the volume as the setting changes. He may attribute a positive or negative benefit to the aspect of user control. Either way, you must identify his feelings to make the best recommendation for hearing instruments with or without user-adjustable volume control.

Remote Control Adjustments

Your client may tell you about friends or family members with remote tools for adjusting the hearing aids. He may voice concerns about misplacing extra parts in the hearing aid system. Or if he has seen this type of instrument used successfully, he may inquire about its benefits. By asking questions and illustrating the use of a remote control, clients will feel more comfortable in sharing their feelings about it. Remote controls are familiar to many television users, but their advantages or disadvantages when applied to hearing aids should still be discussed.

On-Off Switches

Most conventional hearing aids incorporate on-off switches into their design. But many of the more advanced technology hearing aids require that this switch be specifically added or cannot accommodate this option at all. A client's environment plays a large role in determining whether this option should be used during the day. A client working in an intense noise situation without communication requirements (e.g., a factory or job site with heavy equipment) may appreciate the ability to turn the hearing aids off without constantly removing them and reinserting them later. This need should also raise the question of style consideration (i.e., perhaps the hearing aids must fit under earmuffs or ear protective devices without interfering with the use of ear protection). Clinicians must ask about the situations and the background noise present in clients' daily activities to decide if the on-off switch will be a required and desired option.

Multiple Program Options

When discussing a client's daily activities, clinicians can introduce the use of multiple programs. If the client's acoustical settings are very diverse, a hearing system with multiple programs can be designed to accommodate diverse communication needs in multiple settings. For example, an attorney in the courtroom setting may need to hear a witness across a distance of 20 feet or more. The amplification matrix for this setting would differ from the matrix chosen in a group setting. Multiple programs allow the clinician to meet communication needs in a variety of diverse settings. Recently, one hearing aid manufacturer compared the need for multiple programs in hearing with the need for different types of eye wear (e.g., corrective lenses, reading glasses, bifocals, sunglasses, and even ski goggles and scuba masks). Clients are familiar with the different needs for vision and can relate to a discussion of the different needs for hearing including hearing in groups, in noise, across distance, for music, and in automobiles. When discussing the possible different settings, if speech enhancement in noise is the primary concern, perhaps hearing aids containing directional microphones or multiple programs should be recommended. Encourage clients to reflect on the types of communication settings they experience, then prioritize them and weight their relative importance. Then it will become apparent if multiple programs will improve the benefit offered by amplification or if they will complicate the fitting process and therefore reduce the value of amplification.

Digital or Digitally Programmable Circuitry

Clinicians must consider which circuitry will best satisfy a client's expectations for the use of amplification. If the client's range of listening environments is varied and represents complex noise environments, then analog circuitry does not have a good record with user satisfaction in those environments. If noise has been a factor in the failure of previous amplification attempts, then the clinician must consider what circuitry options specifically address this issue. Compression algorithms that allow the clinician access to programming release times may result in increasing the client's comfort in noise. If the client demonstrates a hearing loss configuration that is a steeply sloping, jagged, reversed curve configuration, or unusual configuration, then digital circuitry that allows the most effective frequency shaping may increase the chances for successful amplification. Digitally programmable aids may successfully meet client expectations when programming can be accomplished in one or two channels and when processing strategies are simpler. Although objective data may not yet support it, subjective data do suggest that many listeners function better in noisy environments with digital hearing aids.

SIZE REMAINS A FITTING ISSUE

Although it is important to educate clients to understand differences in technology, most clients readily recognize differences in size. There is a misperception that the smaller the hearing aid, the more advanced the technology. Clients should be educated to appreciate the fallacy of this belief. If the selection of a smaller hearing instrument decreases the performance of that technology for that client, gently, but firmly recommend against it. If the solution chosen will have a shortened life span due to the size option selected, then client must accept responsibility for this decision. Help clients understand that not all size options are appropriate for all hearing losses. Only the clients can decide if the need to improve hearing performance is outweighed by the desired size option. When appropriate, suggest methods to make larger hearing aid style options more cosmetically appealing by color coding the instruments to match hair color, contouring of the shape, and with changes in hairstyles. Clients sometimes apologize for the selection of a hearing aid based on style. *It is insensitive to ignore the fact that hearing instruments can be perceived as the visible signs of aging or handicap. If clients view the hearing instrument as a stigma, it will add to the communication problem and increase the likelihood of failure with amplification.* When stigma is a concern, the visibility of the hearing instruments must be reduced if clients are to succeed. If this compromises performance, the fitting may ultimately fail, but at least it will be the client's choice.

HEARING AID MAINTENANCE ISSUES

When discussing the appearance of the hearing instruments, include the issues of maintenance. Certain types of hearing aids require more care and have higher rates of repair than do others. Clients should know this before the final hearing aid selection is made. Informed clients are responsible for the adequate care of their hearing aids. If you do not enlist their cooperation and responsibility, before the selection, hearing instruments that become unreliable because of improper maintenance, dirt, or cerumen build-up reflect poorly on your professionalism.

PRESENT YOUR BEST RECOMMENDATION

Your best recommendation is based upon removing or alleviating the handicap presented by the client's hearing impairment. To accomplish that goal you must ensure comfort, enhance speech intelligibility and the ability to benefit from the sounds encountered in the client's daily activities. Selling the best technology based upon clinical research, experience, and the most positive outlook for client success is the only viable position in advocating for the most effective hearing solutions. Fitting issues that must be resolved include output limiting, frequency shaping, and flexibility of the circuitry over time. The clinician must first recommend the best choice circuitry for accomplishing these goals. Explain the performance abilities of the technology you have recommended and the relationship of these abilities to the client's expressed needs. Discuss the benefits of your recommendations as they relate to other factors you have discussed with the client; for example the life span, the reliability, and the flexibility of the recommended hearing aids. *Although economics are a part of every hearing aid fitting, individual client priorities—not clinician priorities—should determine where financial resources are allocated.* If it is necessary to explore other options, inform the client of the benefits potentially lost with other types of technology.

Acknowledge the range of other options available, explaining how other choices will alter or detract from satisfying the client's final hearing goals. This is the time to reaffirm your ability to represent the wide range of hearing technology and to reassure the client that you will ensure the best possible informed choice by the client. If the disadvantages in an alternative choice are slight, and the client decides to evaluate a solution with less benefit, involve the client in the responsibility for the decisions. *Unless the client understands the limitations of the chosen technology and comprehends the rationale underlying your recommendations, a recommendation of less than the best technology may place the clinician in a disappointing light as time passes and the client becomes less than satisfied with the hearing results.* For this reason, some clinicians request that clients who demand products and arrangements other than those recommended (i.e., monaural vs. binaural, or CICs vs. ITEs or BTEs) sign a statement acknowledging the difference of opinion.

CONSIDER YOUR ROLE IN FUTURE REHABILITATION

Clinical and scientific evidence suggests that most clients will observe improved hearing benefits with digital signal processors and the advanced technology available in many hybrid systems (Kochkin, 1996). If hearing benefits in complex listening situations are the most important needs for your clients, then you should explain the recommendations as they relate to the solution efficacy that type of technology offers. Base your recommendations on what you know today. Then, establish your position as the knowledge source for new technologies that can be expected to emerge tomorrow. You can offer to update clients on the changes in the hearing industry that will affect future hearing solutions. Subsequent calls (or mailings) to clients become product briefings, rather than sales calls. New knowledge can be incorporated in clients' present fittings during the provision of follow-up service. The knowledgeable consumer relationship is a long-term benefit to the clinician. As new ideas are introduced on the marketplace, clients will return to the clinician/counselor for advice on integrating new ideas or systems into their current hearing solutions. The long-term relationships we establish encourage clients to view us as vendors of problem solving techniques. Selling hearing solutions and systems based on available technology rather than selling today's "best" hearing aids places clinicians in the best counseling position. *There is no need to champion a particular device if your goal is to champion technology to meet hearing needs. Selling the knowledge of technology advances transitions the profession of audiology from the undesirable selling of a "fix" or product, to the marketing of choices for lifestyle change.* And this transition cannot help but dramatically affect the evolving field of hearing health care systems.

To keep pace with changing developments in hardware, we need to reconsider programs based on possession of the current solution, not necessarily ownership. Ownership is a concept tied to the generations before the Baby Boomers. Experience is the more contemporary expectation. As with the "your ware" program mentioned earlier, leasing programs allow the Baby Boomer generation to expect the use of the best: the best cars, the best vacation homes, the best personal accessories, for as long as they care to use them. In designing programs based on leasing expectations, the relationship with the provider becomes more important and outlives the product expectations of the user. Perhaps future users of amplification will view the need for a hearing experience guided by audiology professionals rather than the ownership of hearing aids. These changes could affect our ultimate role in the hearing health care system and provide an opportunity to move the marketing of knowledge systems to a central point in the hearing health care delivery system. *Providers in today's marketplace must explore their competencies and prepare to transition their skills to match not only clients' hearing needs, but also the needs of tomorrow's delivery systems.* Changing competencies require audiology professionals to improve our basic counseling skills and to market our abilities to assist clients in improving their lifestyles with the appropriate selection of hearing aid technology. By establishing client-centered relationships, we may refocus our clients on the purchase of professional competencies. The client-centered relationship empowers hearing professionals to market the fitting of hearing solutions, not just the purchase of hearing devices, thus re-creating the central role of professionals in the selection and fitting of hearing aid technology.

SUMMARY AND TIPS FOR ESTABLISHING CLIENT-CENTERED RELATIONSHIPS

The development of the client-centered relationship allows the hearing professional to market information and not hearing devices. This crucial shift in the consumer's perception of the role of the hearing professional substantially increases the viability of the individual hearing health care practice. The steps in establishing client-centered relationships involve the entire hearing health care team, the marketing of hearing aids, and the establishment of client oriented policies and procedures.

1. Market activities to promote your practice as a consumer-safe source for hearing information.
2. Train your entire administrative team to set the tone when the consumer first contacts your office.
3. Design the first appointment to allow the consumer to experience your practice with minimal risk.
   a. Offer a relaxed, friendly environment.
   b. Gather diagnostic information efficiently and courteously.
   c. Counsel clients to share their experiences with hearing loss and aids.
4. Match technology to the client's statements of hearing needs.
   a. Identify key features or options based upon counseling to determine the client's statement of needs.
   b. Match technology options to fulfill the client's expectations of benefit based upon agreed upon outcomes.
5. Maintain ongoing relationships with clients to assure the continued quality of the hearing aid fitting.
   a. Provide product briefings and information on new developments in technology.
   b. Provide product briefings and information on assistive listening devices.
   c. Become the source for companion products that improve changing lifestyles.

REFERENCES

Kochkin, S. (1996). Customer satisfaction and subjective benefit with high performance hearing aids. *The Hearing Review. 3,* (12), 16, 18, 22–24, 26.
Strom, K. (1998). The 1997 hearing instrument market—The dispensers' perspective. *The Hearing Review. 5*(6), 4.

Historically, many audiologists have had a difficult time in putting a price on and requiring fees for their services, be they diagnostic or rehabilitative. The use of the term "selling" carries a repugnant connotation to some audiologists. Less than 25 years ago audiologists could actually lose their license if they "sold" hearing aids for a profit. The reality, as emphasized throughout this book, is that we are indeed "selling"; but rather than selling a product, *per se, we are selling the* process *of hearing. Hearing aids are one of the most vital components comprising the process (speechreading, controlling the acoustic environment, learning methods to "fill in the gaps," etc., are among the others). If we don't convince patients to wear hearing aids, we are not fulfilling our obligation to provide them with every available opportunity to maximize their hearing abilities.*

Because audiology is taking on a more professional aura every day, it behooves us to get a better grasp on the entrepreneurial aspect of the profession. As trained scientists, many of us are uncomfortable with this necessary but sometimes uncomfortable portion of our profession. As mentioned in Chapter 1, "sales" is not a dirty word, as long as the procedures are performed in a manner and intent that is consistent with the best needs of the patient. In Chapter 6, Rennae Pickert describes procedures and methods that have been derived from "sales" practices. Therefore, the terms "sales," "salesperson," "client," and "customer" are used in this context.

The ideas in this chapter were derived from the author's personal experience as manager of a successful multiple-office private practice. Although not all of the concepts proposed are applicable to every dispensing facility, the majority of these suggestions can be implemented by most practices.

6

How to Sell Hearing Professionally

■ **Rennae Pickert, M.S.** ■

The success of a hearing instrument practice, not unlike most other retail businesses, depends on a three-part formula. The strategy presented here can be a blueprint for a hearing aid dispensing business plan and, if utilized, can result in financial growth and produce an increased number of patients who will attest to enjoying a better quality of life. The formula is based on:

Getting patients in the door + Getting patients to purchase the products + Getting products to "stick" (e.g., avoiding returns) = *Success*

Each segment of this formula requires good counseling, listening, and selling techniques in order for it to be implemented successfully.

Historically, hearing instrument specialists have directed their focus mainly on technological training including:

■ What type of hearing loss is it (e.g., sensorineural or conductive)?

- What type of output limiting should I use (e.g., input vs. output, linear or wide dynamic range compression)?
- What type of sound processing (e.g., digital or analog)?
- What style of device (e.g., behind-the-ear or completely-in-the-canal)?

Countless hours of continuing education are required to keep abreast of the technological advances introduced by manufacturers today. We have evolved from basic offices supplied with an acoustical enclosure and one modification wheel to offices equipped with computers, programmers, elaborate modification equipment, and new software updates that arrive almost weekly. The focus has been on technology. This is good, but it has also left many hearing instrument specialists lacking in the field of business training. Few training programs spend time on learning and understanding the various aspects of sales, marketing, and counseling. Consequently, as a profession, we are not reaching the numbers of patients who need our help, as evidenced by poor market penetration of hearing aid sales. Not only is there a void in business knowledge and training, but many hearing instrument specialists are uncomfortable with the concepts underlying sales and marketing. Somewhere along the line, the "selling" of hearing instruments developed a negative connotation in the minds of many specialists. This may be because:

- The educational content provided in our training programs has limited our roles to being only *service* providers.
- We may feel that a monetary value should not be attached to the services we provide.
- We may feel like we do not deserve to make a profit.
- There may be a lack of confidence in the benefit that patients will receive from our instruments.
- We may be afraid of rejection.
- We may simply lack the skills necessary to sell and market our businesses effectively.

In the United States alone, there are about 28 million people who have some degree of hearing loss. Out of this 28 million, it is estimated that only about 6 million, or approximately 20%, wear amplification. This leaves 80% of the population that is hearing impaired lacking instrumentation *necessary* to communicate effectively. This percentage is much less than other *luxury product categories,* such as cellular phones and personal computers. Why is the number of patients resisting our help so high? Possible reasons include:

- Patients who are hearing impaired lack confidence in what hearing instruments can do because of media reports or unsuccessful prior fittings on family members, friends, or even themselves.
- Patients may be unaware of their problem. They may blame others and deny the consequences of their hearing loss.
- They may be unaware of the newest advances in technology and cosmetics.
- There may be insufficient financial resources. If the money is not available, the hearing problem may have a low financial priority.
- They may have had bad experiences with a hearing instrument specialist who was unskilled in appropriate counseling and fitting approaches.
- They may have been unexposed to effective advertising or exposed to only "tacky, low-budget" advertising, thus reinforcing their skepticism.

Hearing instrument specialists need to have a new mission. We need to stop worrying about the local competition in our area. Our competition is the 22 million people who are not wearing amplification. These unserved people are missing out on the potential of enhanced communication that is important to maintaining a good quality of life. Some are lonely, depressed, aging, isolated, and possibly a burden to family members and friends. It is our task to help them hear to the best of their ability. Through our experience, we have found that we can accomplish this goal by following the formula presented earlier (i.e., first, getting them in the door; second, getting them to purchase the appropriate products; and third, getting them to keep and wear the products). The end results are (1) happy patients, (2) happy friends and family members, and (3) a successful and profitable hearing instrument practice. This is our opportunity to make a difference. Our mission may not be accomplished unless we learn and implement business, marketing, and counseling skills *and* feel good about what we are doing!

Six years ago, my company was a small organization, consisting of one full-time office and one part-time office. We employed two full-time receptionists and three part-time dispensing audiologists. It was commonplace at that time to service an average of 8 patients per day. Six years ago, we implemented the three-part formula and now staff 16 employees, have five full-time offices, service approximately 50 patients per day, and have increased our gross sales by 300%. We developed a business plan that systematically helps us accomplish the goals of getting the patients in the door, getting them to purchase, and getting them to keep and wear the products purchased. This plan has dictated many laborious changes over the years and is continuously being improved. We believe we owe our success to the formula.

GETTING PATIENTS IN THE DOOR

Image

It is intuitively obvious to say that, before you can help patients hear or help your practice grow, you must get the patients in the door. This step may vary in difficulty depending on your type of facility. Medical practices may have less difficulty if referring physicians are somewhat aggressive in recognizing the need for and recommending amplification. Retail facilities, on the other end of the spectrum, must work diligently for each patient who walks through the door. To increase the number of prospective patients seen, regardless of the type of facility, your company must be represented with a professional image.

My company started the process of changing its image with a name and location change. The old company name (Dallas Audiological Services) seemed to be difficult for patients to say, tough for patients to hear on the telephone, and somewhat confusing, sadly enough, regarding the meaning of "Audiological." We believed that a consumer-oriented name would increase awareness of our practice. By changing our name to "Sound Hearing Solutions," we believe that we have accomplished this goal because it implies a problem-solving theme to patients. Choosing a new location has contributed to our image change even more dramatically. Our higher volume office is easily visible from the street, located next to a busy restaurant in a shopping center that targets the elderly population, and has ample parking available.

The goal in image changing is to leave patients with a memory of the best buying experience they have ever had.

- It is important to have a nice decor that is clean and different, with soothing music in the waiting room and even outside the office.
- Patients need to see signs of confidence in the office (e.g., professional photos of employees, awards, certificates, testimonials, books, and photos of happy patients).
- Our chart system has been converted into a visible one that lines the office walls to demonstrate our longevity and stability to patients.
- It is a nice gesture to have coffee and baked goods in the waiting room to make patients feel welcome.
- Patients need to see that the office is organized and updated. Computers in the office for office management and hearing instrument fittings contribute to the desired image.
- Office management systems help keep protocols in place and prevent mistakes (e.g., mistaken appointment scheduling) from destroying your image.

Presenting patients with a good image of the organization heightens their receptivity of the forthcoming information they will hear about their hearing loss and recommendations for remediation.

Advertising is necessary to help increase the number of potential hearing instrument wearers seen. Potential candidates must see that there are new developments in technology and cosmetics, and they must increase their awareness of the signs of hearing loss. Advertising done with a professional style will help combat the negative information that patients may absorb from the media and other sources. A portion of gross sales should be spent on consistent and frequent advertising that will eventually pay for itself and contribute to overall growth. Six years ago, my company invested zero dollars in advertising. We now dedicate approximately 13% of our gross income to advertising. We advertise using a combination of media including newspaper, direct mail, television, radio, and newsletters to current patients. A successful marketing piece for us has been "The Consumer Guide to Hearing Aids" produced by our advertising agent, Wilson and Co., Ft. Worth, TX. This book is advertised in the area newspaper as a free information booklet on amplification (see Figure 6–1). Not only is this booklet useful to patients, but it allows their names to become a part of our client base for future mailings. We have found it to be cost effective to hire an advertising agency that specializes in hearing instruments to develop a marketing plan and to design our ads.

It is important to develop other lead generators within the practice that can augment the other areas of advertising used in your practice. The best way to identify and target potential patients is through your office management system. With this, you can create lists of:

- patients who have older instruments,
- patients who did not purchase during the initial visit,
- patients with specific configurations of hearing loss,
- patients needing warranty checks,
- battery club participants,
- birthdays of patients.

Information about new technology, consumer seminars, newsletters, and birthday cards can be sent to these patients. Most patients enjoy meaningful contacts from your office on a routine basis. Eventually, they will be back in the office seeking better hearing solutions. Don't forget to reward your patients for their referrals. This can be one of your strongest referral sources if everyone in the practice is doing the best job possible.

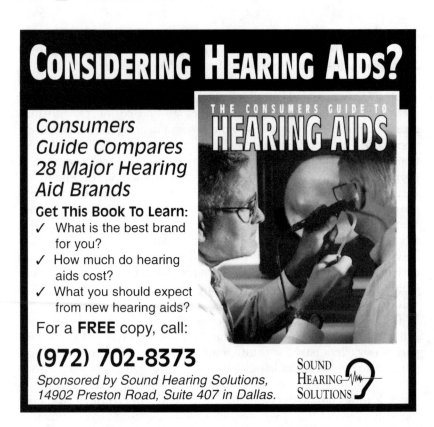

Figure 6–1. Advertisement for "The Consumer Guide to Hearing Aids."

Image equals confidence. If a good image foundation has been laid in the mind of patients, they will believe what you have to tell them about their hearing and trust your recommendation for amplification. This industry, historically, has created reasons for skepticism in potential patients. Unfortunately, skepticism can interfere with the quality of life of patients and their families and also reduce the success we experience in private practice. Establishing a good image to patients you have attracted into the office or to those considering amplification is the door that must open before the rest of your goals can be reached.

GETTING PATIENTS TO PURCHASE HEARING PRODUCTS

Typically, in the hearing instrument industry, only limited success is achieved unless patients purchase products. If the hearing instrument specialist is not able to convince the patient that hearing instruments are necessary vehicles for improving his hearing problems, then everyone loses. The patient leaves the office with the same hearing loss and communication problems that he entered with; the specialist has lost the chance to improve the patient's quality of life; and from a business standpoint, a sale has been lost. All the time, money, and training spent getting the patient in the door has accomplished nothing. Ultimately, when a patient decides not to purchase, he will either (a) continue to be unhappy and belong to the group of about 22 million people who do not wear hearing instruments, (b) purchase instruments from another facility, or (c) inform other potential customers that your company may not be the one to work with. In any case, the entire selling process should be examined to determine where changes need to be made.

- Did the specialist not gain the patient's trust?
- Did the specialist not explain the hearing loss in such a way that the patient realized he had a hearing problem?
- Was the presentation of hearing instruments too confusing or not convincing?
- Did the specialist lack the counseling skills to analyze the needs and goals of the patient?
- Did the specialist lack the skills to help the patient make the right decision?
- Did the specialist simply not feel comfortable with "selling"?

If hearing instrument specialists don't feel comfortable with "selling" in general, it will affect all components of the hearing device process including the interview, hearing evaluation, explanation of the loss and hearing instrument technology, goal setting, gaining confidence, and decision making. There is a high probability that a primary reason for this discomfort is that specialists in our industry do not realize that there is a difference between "nonprofessional" and "professional" selling. The key word here is "professional." This is the degree to which salespersons identify patients' needs and respond to them. It is the exact opposite of manipulating patients to purchase products or services they did not need or that were not appropriate for them. *Professional selling involves professionals having a realistic understanding of patients' needs; realistically communicating the value of products; and having confidence in themselves, their products, and their organizations.* It also involves the effective use of marketing and helping patients to make informed decisions.

In our office, professional selling is a multidimensional process that is omnipresent throughout every activity that occurs. The entire organization is excited about the chance to *sell* better hearing. Selling occurs from the moment patients make their initial telephone call through the years of following up on the instrument fitting. Selling occurs during informational telephone calls, appointment setting, calming irate patients, battery sales, repairs, product returns, hearing aid evaluations and consultations, product purchases, and follow-up visits. Every level of this process must be aligned for success to be achieved.

The basis for effective selling is to have an effective sales team. This team includes not only those who sell the products directly (i.e., the hearing instrument specialists), but also those who sell indirectly, the front office staff. These individuals hold a vitally important position in the entire sales process. They are the contact patients have to the office. Immediately, during that first telephone call or when walking in the door, an image of the practice is formed. The front office staff must be skillful at turning a telephone inquiry into an appointment and comforting upset patients with solutions. These skills will directly affect the success of a practice. They have a direct impact on the bottom line and on the hearing help that patients receive.

A recent study was conducted by Age Wave Enterprises, San Francisco, to determine the level of competence with which the front office staff at audiology offices around the country handled patients' phone calls, questions about hearing in general, and their ability to encourage callers to schedule appointments. The study involved recording the various front office staff's responses to a "mystery shopper" inquiring about hearing instruments. The results of the study concluded that, generally, front office staffs seemed to know little about the industry and seemed to have poor customer service and sales skills. Our front office staff has undergone a training program called "AAA Frontline Office Training Kit: Initiating the Journey." This kit, available through the American Academy of Audiology, contains information on effectively communicating with patients and important information on audiology and hearing health. The kit, which consists of a videotape, an audiotape, reference cards, and a workbook, has been effective in preparing our front office staff to deal with patients. It is also important for the front office staff to keep an ongoing count of telephone inquiries, what the appropriate referral sources were, and the percentage of those who actually scheduled an appointment. In our office, these figures are reviewed monthly in order to focus on areas for improvement. Role-playing has also proven to be an effective exercise for our front office staff.

The entire sales team must possess certain skills and attributes to be effective in their position. They must have:

- **Positive attitudes.** The entire sales team must feel good about the selling process. They must believe that through sales they are helping patients to hear better. They must want to take every opportunity to help patients make decisions, from scheduling appointments to purchasing hearing instruments. It may be necessary to evaluate the personality types of existing team members (see Chapter 3) and make changes in personnel in order to maximize each position. Each opportunity that is missed for scheduling an appointment, selling products, or avoiding a return not only costs the practice money, but also contributes to the population of unaided patients.

- **Product knowledge.** Every staff member must possess current and in-depth knowledge of all products, services, warranties, and procedures. As a result of increased advertising and access to product information through the Internet, our patients have become more informed. The inquiries have become more technical and require increased product understanding. Consumers spend more time on information gathering and comparing, and they develop confidence in a practice that proves to be knowledgeable. The entire staff must participate in continuing education and manufacturer training to be prepared for this level of patient.

- **People knowledge.** Each patient must be treated as a unique individual. One patient's needs may be completely different than those of another. The entire staff must possess the ability to "power listen," which involves an ability to hear what the patient is *really* saying. What a patient says and what he really means may be diametrically opposed. Patients must feel that each team member is receptive to their needs. Professional in-office training on personality types and counseling techniques is helpful in providing your staff with tools to increase people knowledge. These matters are discussed in Chapters 2 and 3.

- **Selling skills.** An organized sales plan commencing with gathering information and continuing through closing the sale will lead to "professional selling." Selling skills must extend throughout the entire relationship with a patient, even after the purchase has been made. Professional selling is centered around a six-step multisensory *value* selling process. This is a process of determining a patient's needs, lifestyle, finances, goals, and desires in order to determine the appropriate products for his profile. The process includes promoting the impact that these products and your services will have on the patient's needs. You must be able to satisfy the products/services needs of the patient, as well as his psychological needs. The key to implementing this process successfully is communication. The following six basic steps constitute this process and involve the entire office staff:

1. *Attracting the patient's immediate and favorable attention* starts with the image he develops about your practice from the initial contact that is made. The patient's attention will be favorable if he believes the office is a successful one. The office must look professional and the staff must act professionally. All staff members should wear name tags including their first name. Patients should be greeted pleasantly by the receptionist. The staff should try to remember important personal details about all patients and ask about them periodically (e.g., "How was your trip to France?" "How is your grandson's soccer team?" etc.). Attracting favorable attention begins in the front office area and continues into the fitting/examination room.

2. *Determining a patient's needs* is an ongoing process originating during the initial telephone inquiry, continuing throughout the evaluation, and even through postfitting appointments. Establishing a patient's needs requires in-depth questioning, probing, interaction, and reading between the lines. It is important to determine what the patient thinks he is in your office for, what his motivation level is, and what his goals are. Subjective information can be gathered during the initial interview with the patient and his significant others. This interview will be more effectively orchestrated by collecting written information prior to the visit. Our patient information form (see Appendix 6-A) includes questions regarding level of motivation and the hierarchy of important features. It has been an effective tool to help understand patients' true feelings toward amplification. To make appropriate recommendations regarding products and technology, the specialist must determine the patient's lifestyle and where he is experiencing difficulty. The Listening Abilities Questionnaire (see Appendix 6-B) is completed in our office to help profile patients. Determining the patient's goals for amplification is critical to the entire evaluation process. The goals, once determined, should be ranked in order of importance (e.g., using the COSI as seen in Appendix 6-C) and used as a benchmark for progress during the postfitting process. Specialists must evaluate what patients are really saying when "complaints" about hearing instruments are reported. These complaints need to be related back to the original goals (e.g., established in the COSI) to determine if action needs to be taken or if it is counseling that is necessary. Unrealistic goals should be indicators for potential failures. Recognizing these goals will help identify patients who may need to consider amplification at a later

date, but who may need alternatives in the meantime. Physical and mental constraints must be identified through observation and factored into the recommendations for such patients.

3. *Describing the benefits the patient should expect from amplification* requires that the specialist tailors her presentation of information to the educational level of the patient to maximize the outcome of the consultation. For suggestions, refer to Chapter 4. Being receptive to comments, questions, and body language will help determine the patient's level of understanding and should indicate the direction that the specialist should go with the conversation. The audiogram should be discussed in relationship to the patient's original communication problems. The Audibility Index (see Appendix 6-D) is used in our office to demonstrate what percentage of speech understanding is affected by the particular hearing impairment. This index can be adapted to fit the educational level of patients. If patients appear to be in denial, the problems they are having with their hearing loss can easily be demonstrated (e.g., by presenting a high-frequency sound without any visual cues). This is most effective if a loved one is present and can verify the sound. Describe in general how amplification should change what has just been observed.

4. *Providing enough facts and features about products and services* is vital. Professional selling can only continue if the presentation of products is organized and clear. Specialists must maintain the attention of patients in order for them to feel confident with purchasing products. If the proper counseling tools have been used thus far and patients' needs, goals, wants, and lifestyles have been determined, then this step in the process should be impressive. All patients with hearing loss should observe a product demonstration. They should be able to listen to what a difference hearing instruments can make. *It is important to let patients listen to premier technology, in spite of any cost concerns. All patients deserve to hear what their hearing potential can be.* If "cost" is listed as a patient's number one priority, it could mean that the patient can afford the best technology, but does not want to spend the money. Your recommendation for particular instruments can then be altered if this level of technology is out of his price range. Sales aids can clarify technical aspects of the demonstration. We use a flip chart in each fitting room containing diagrams of sound waves, ear anatomy, effects of amplification on hearing loss, styles of hearing instruments, feedback loop, and digital sound processing. It is important not to confuse the patient by describing every product on the market. Too many choices leave patients confused and will give

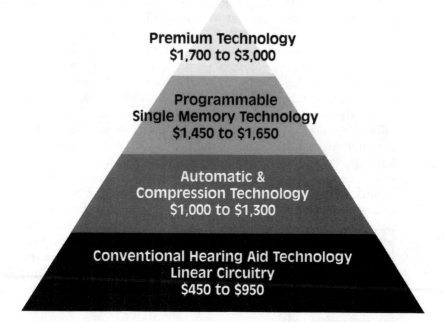

Figure 6–2. Product Pyramid (developed by Wilson and Company, Inc.).

them more reasons to "go home and think about it." Hearing specialists are, after all, the specialists and should be able to guide patients in the appropriate direction. We use a product pyramid, developed by Wilson and Company, Inc. (see Figure 6–2), that categorizes hearing instruments by cost and technology. This can be used to determine in which price category a patient may fit. The recommendation would then be the most appropriate instruments in that category.

5. *Overcoming objections, concerns, and misunderstandings* requires that hearing specialists use counseling skills to determine the basis for the objections of patients. If objections, concerns, and misunderstandings aren't overcome, then patients will not purchase hearing instruments. They will not be helped, nor will you. What a patient says may be a result of a personality trait that triggers objections (see Chapter 3). Patients may be resistant to any change, reluctant to making any decision, want to bargain for a better deal, want to test the hearing specialist's knowledge, in denial, or simply not be psychologically ready. Could the specialist have talked over the patient's head, failed to establish rapport with the patient

before the presentation, or failed to identify the patient's true needs, therefore stressing the wrong benefit? *Objections should be welcomed and considered a clue to indicate what part of the presentation was not clear.* This will provide the specialist with a chance to concentrate on those areas. Respecting a patient's objections shows that you care. A patient's emotional discomfort will be reduced if he is allowed to talk. Listening helps the specialist identify what is important to the patient. Qualify objections by stating what you think you hear from the patient. Verify the objection, pause, and listen more. Empathize with patients by acknowledging their concerns. Never contradict concerns of patients, and do not try to argue with them using "Yes, but." This tells them that they are wrong and will put them on the defense. Rephrase the objection and convert it into a question (e.g., "So, are you concerned that these hearing aids will be too visible?"). This process will keep patients off the defense and will avoid argumentative responses. Offer evidence. We use the "feel, felt, found" approach in our office. For example, if patients are concerned that behind-the-ear hearing instruments will be too visible, we would respond in the following manner. "I know how you *feel*. Many of our patients have *felt* the same way. But, when they have worn the instruments with a tiny earmold and with the instruments hiding under their hair, they have *found* that no one has even been able to see them." Additional benefits of the particular product should then be added (e.g., durability, less occlusion, less feedback, more power, etc.). Look for signs that help you determine the patient's level of agreement, such as head nodding, eye widening, or brow placement. Always be prepared for the patient's objections. Knowledgeable answers should be formulated in preparation for common objections.

6. *Closing the sale* is, of course, essential. To help the patient improve his quality of life, he must make the purchase. As a professional salesperson, you must help him make a decision and feel comfortable with his commitment for action. A good closer is a skilled closer. Specific steps must be taken to avoid the situation turning into one of the following:

a. "hard close," which turns the patient off, resulting in a non-purchase,

b. "selling beyond the close," which involves the salesperson talking too much and consequently losing the patient's interest,

c. "no close," in which the salesperson makes no effort to take the order, and the patient is put in the position to end the session without purchasing.

A professional salesperson is constantly looking for "buying signals," such as picking up the contract, open hands, nonverbal communication, difficulty deciding between two products, or inquiries about the financial arrangements. Timing and skill is everything in closing a sale professionally. If the closing is unsuccessful, the patient will rejoin the 22 million people in the United States without amplification or he will purchase from a competitor who *can* professionally close the sale. Depending on what you have learned thus far from the patient, there are several ways to close a sale:

- *The Experimental Close* allows the salesperson a chance to evaluate the patient's commitment on a minor point. From his response, it can be determined if more information is needed or if the sale is ready to close. For example, "How do you feel about this product in the behind-the-ear style?" Several experimental closes may be used during the evaluation procedure to determine readiness to the actual close.
- *The Presumptive Close* involves assuming the patient is going to purchase. This is used based on the patient's reception to the product during several experimental closes. A key word that can be used in the experimental close is "when" or phrases referring to timing. For example, "When do you want these hearing instruments delivered?" or "Is this something you want to get started with today?" If the response to this close is negative, it gives the salesperson a chance to determine what information is needed to overcome the objection.
- *The Choice Close* is similar to the experimental close, but is used after the patient shows definite receptivity to the product. Questions such as, "Which instruments do you feel you would be happiest with?" are used with this approach.
- *The Action Close* occurs when the professional salesperson identifies a high level of receptivity from the patient and initiates an action to bring about the close. The salesperson must disclose the action necessary to get started. For example, "All we need to do today is to make earmold impressions and sign the purchase agreement." This close provides a tool to help the patient make up his mind.
- *The Enticement Close* offers the patient an incentive to make the purchase now rather than putting it off. For example, "Mrs. Jones, you'll be happy to know that every product ordered this week has a free second year's warranty included in the price." This close is to be used only when all others have failed. People enjoy getting something extra and can be motivated toward a decision if they believe it is a limited offer.
- *The Summary Close* is typically used in combination with the action close. Summarize the benefits that were discussed and observed dur-

ing the evaluation, then talk about the next logical step. For example, "Now that you have observed how these digital hearing instruments have improved your comfort in background noise, all we need to do is to make earmold impressions and sign the purchase agreement."

■ *The Two Step Close* begins with assessing an opinion. For example, "So, how do you feel about what these hearing instruments can do for your problems?" If the answer is unfavorable, it gives the salesperson a chance to overcome the patient's objection with more information. If the response is positive, then proceed to the next step, closing on a recommendation. "What I'd like to recommend today is that we get earmold impressions and order a set of . . ."

Throughout the entire process dispensers must demonstrate *value* to patients. If patients believe they will be buying true value, then the balance scale will be tipped toward making the purchase. Most major objections are centered around price, psychological resistance to making a change, and risk. These objections must be overcome for patients to believe they are buying value.

Selling the value of your products and services will help overcome any pricing issue. Hearing specialists must sell the quality of the personnel, superior service, and a proven track record of happy customers. A patient must be told that price is relative when a competitor is mentioned. Make sure he understands everything he is getting for the price from your company. Price is only one part of the overall cost of a product. You must find out to what part of the "price" the patient is referring. Does he believe the price is too high? Is the product not worth the money? Does he believe he can get the same product from another establishment at a lesser price? Or, does he simply not have the funds? At this point, it is important to reexamine the goals he originally had for the hearing instruments and find out which one of these goals he is willing to give up in order to stay in his price range. The patient will then associate price with value. Become "price proud." You must feel that the value is worth the price. Selling value justifies the price.

Psychological resistance to making a decision sometimes carries greater weight than price. Good counseling and listening skills can help reveal where this resistance is based. Help patients evaluate their situation and discover a reason or value for making a change. Using lead phrases (e.g., "Let me ask you a question") can help reduce resistance to change.

Finally, risk can be the most significant event in the buying process. Patients typically think about what they will lose by making a bad decision. Professional salespersons have documentation that proves their company stands behind their promises in both products and services. Ask patients what they need from you to be more comfortable about making this decision. An important thing to remember is that, although patients may use price as their main objection, it may be risk or psychological resistance that is keeping them from moving forward with a decision.

To execute professional selling in your office, the staff must be involved in extensive training, role-playing, lectures, modeling, and observation of numerous successful sales sessions. The entire process must be successful for patients to feel comfortable with making a decision. If the process is done incorrectly, it will only add to the stereotype that is prevalent in the hearing instrument industry today. The entire staff must feel comfortable with sales for this to be perceived by patients as natural. If a staff member is uncomfortable, it is likely that she will be unable to learn the process. Personnel changes in our company over the last 6 years have dramatically contributed to our growth. We now employ only people with good communication skills and good attitudes who are good listeners and who are excited about selling. Not only has our practice prospered, but our patients have ultimately benefited from the changes we have made. Our patients have had exciting buying experiences and feel good about our approach. This translates into excitement about the help they can receive from our products and services.

GETTING PATIENTS TO KEEP THE INSTRUMENTS

A feeling of accomplishment and success is typically manifested in a hearing instrument specialist's mind when the patient agrees to go forward with the fitting of the product. It can feel like a wave of relief, excitement, and satisfaction. It is a verification that the patient approved of the image of the office, the expertise of the specialist, and the format of the product presentation. All of the time, money, and effort spent to achieve an appointment with this patient has paid off. Professional selling has taken place.

More detrimental to patients and to our industry than an unprofessional sales experience is, however, to cease the professionalism when the dotted line is signed. The sale, and more important, the aural rehabilitation program, does not end with the purchase of hearing aids. Sales personnel must realize that a patient can leave the office with a comfortable feeling that doesn't last. *The time lapse between the purchase of the instruments and the fitting may be filled with skeptical or critical comments from the patient's family or friends.* The purchase price of the instruments may now seem extravagant when unexpected financial situations arise. Derogatory reports regarding hearing instruments may appear in the media. The communication problems that precipitated the purchase may now seem insignificant. Any or all of these experiences may trigger the feeling of "buyer's remorse" and will ultimately reduce the patient's motivation level for success with the instruments. A patient who remains enthused about the purchase can also lose his enthusiasm during the postfitting period. In either case, our biggest fear can ring true. If professional selling does not continue throughout the entire relationship with each patient, the hearing instruments may be returned for credit, and the patient may not receive the potential benefits from amplification or further rehabilitation for enhanced communication.

Hearing instrument returns are a disappointing facet of our industry. Because the law allows it, many patients enter the purchase with a "temporary" commitment. These people are essentially "lending us their money" for 30 days. They are the skeptical, unmotivated, proving-a-point type of patient. These are the patients who are constantly concerned with the amount of time that remains on their trial period. They are the ones who have a self-fulfilling prophecy of failure with hearing instruments. They are our most difficult patients. The other type of patient truly wants to succeed and does try to give the instruments the benefit of the doubt. The likelihood of this type of patient returning the instruments is reduced if true benefit is experienced.

If our goal is to help the hearing impaired, we must, as painful as it may seem, examine every single case in which hearing instruments have been returned for credit. We must then formulate a strategy to reduce these numbers. We have implemented a program in our office that has dramatically reduced the number of hearing instrument returns over the past year. This program is based on the information gathered by compiling and analyzing the "profile" data (see Appendix 6-E) derived from patients returning hearing aids.

Getting the patient to keep the purchased hearing instrument begins at the first appointment with image and confidence building. The most important step in this procedure is to sell the most appropriate instruments to the patient in the beginning. Establishing goals at the onset is critical to making the right recommendation. Listening to what the patient is "really" saying will save time and avoid emotional distress. A patient may originally say that cosmetics are not important to him, when in reality instruments that are visible make him feel self-conscious and old. This will interfere with his appreciation of the hearing benefit he is truly experiencing and will result in a return. A patient may convince the specialist that the only style of instruments he is willing to wear are those that, in effect, are inappropriate for his loss.

This fitting will likely not be successful and will also result in a return. If lack of money forces a patient to purchase inferior technology, he must fully understand the limitations of the instruments. If he expects to pay less and experience more, he will be disappointed and return the instruments.

Avoid overzealous selling. The person scheduling the appointment or the specialist working with the patient may be so excited about the technology that the patient will "hear" unrealistic claims about its performance. When a patient's expectations are too high, he can only be disappointed. Be honest. Warn him up front of the difference he may experience with his own voice, occlusion, telephone, and wind noise. If he expects these things, he won't be surprised. He must understand that these are still hearing "aids" and will only help hearing problems, not cure them. *Don't make promises the hearing instruments can't keep.* Disappointment can only lead to returns for credit and unhappy patients.

Do not use the 30-day trial period as a no-risk maneuver to close the sale. A trial period is mandated by most state laws and serves as a consumer protection. Although state laws vary, patients must be told that they have the right to return products if they are not satisfied with them. This is not to say, however, that patients should be encouraged to "just try the hearing aids; you have nothing to lose." This approach may alert the patient that he may not like the hearing instruments. He may then expect to fail. Comments such as, "What do you have to lose?" should be avoided. If a person feels he has nothing to lose by returning the hearing aids, he may be too quick to give up. Although the patient knows that he has the right to return the instruments within 30 days, this period may be better referred to as the 30-day adjustment period. Although somewhat controversial, and subject to local laws, some dispensers prefer to charge patients a trial fee or restocking lab fee.

Be selective. Certain patients should not be fitted. When a patient is in complete denial, believes he has no problem, and is in your office only because his wife dragged him there, then the chance of helping him through amplification alone is slim. If, during a product demonstration, a patient reports he can hear no difference, he may not be ready for hearing instruments. Good counseling and power listening should help identify this type of patient. Successfully closing this sale will accomplish nothing and will usually result in failure in the end. *Good professionals must take this opportunity to offer other aspects of the rehabilitation package to patients and their families at this time that could ultimately prepare them to try amplification in the future.*

The actual fitting process must include the time from when the patient orders the hearing instruments throughout all the postfitting appointments. Successful fittings require a multidimensional approach involving the entire office staff. A thorough fitting regimen has been implemented in our office since 1994 and is an integral part of our success. This has contributed to the 15% decrease of hearing instrument returns over the last 6 years. This procedure is centered around customer service and focuses on continuous patient contact.

Before the hearing instrument dispensing date, it is critical for the front office staff to ensure that all of the necessary components are in the office and are in working order. It is our goal to minimize the waiting time following the order. The telephone call should not be made unless an appointment is available the next day. The hearing instrument dispensing should be a pleasant and informative experience for a patient. He is embarking on an emotional and expensive experience, and it is our job to comfort him in this venture. The fitting room should be ready when the patient walks in. Any necessary data entry into the computer or necessary paperwork should have been completed before his arrival. The new instruments should be displayed in such a way that they look valuable in the patient's mind. The room should be clean with ample lighting and magnifiers available. All of the hesitation the patient may have been feeling should be minimized as the process unfolds.

Once the instruments have been fitted to the patient, the programming portion begins. The instruments are programmed in both quiet and adverse environments. Verification of benefit is documented through real-ear and functional-gain measurements. Maintenance and insertion instructions are illustrated with the assistance of a flip chart of pictorial representations of each procedure. A checklist is completed in the presence of the patient indicating details discussed in the session. A copy of this list should be given to the patient for his files. The patient, before leaving the office, must demonstrate mastery of insertion and maintenance. All patients leave our office with a Hearing Instrument Dispensing folder that contains information regarding troubleshooting, expectations, battery specials, and telephone use. A daily wearing schedule based on a hierarchy of listening environments and a personal diary are given to patients with the assurance that these will be reviewed in each follow-up session.

It is important to review the patient's goals that were established in the initial evaluation and use these goals on a weekly basis to measure progress. Counseling all patients regarding the initial problems they will experience with hearing instruments is critical to acceptance during the first few weeks. Remind patients of the limitations of even the most sophisticated technology *before* their departure to keep their expectations realistic. If, for example, a patient has been alerted about the sound of newspaper rattling, his own voice, occlusion, and problems on the telephone, reaction to these situations will be less likely to result in a return of the instruments.

Weekly follow-up visits are scheduled in our office as patients leave the office. Our customer service department makes a follow-up telephone call after each appointment to offer encouragement and evaluate the changes made at that visit. If needed, patients are scheduled immediately to take care of any acute problems. The COSI is used weekly to evaluate progress toward achieving the original goals. Complaints about a hearing instrument during postfitting visits unrelated to original goals can be a sign that a patient is unwilling to succeed. Using the COSI to stay on track can minimize random complaints and can help the specialist determine the appropriate direction. During follow-up visits, listen to the patient. Evaluate complaints objectively, if possible. Mistakes can be made when the specialist immediately responds with counseling about the adjustment process when there truly is a problem with the instrument. Assure patients that you, too, have high goals for the instruments. Know when to counsel and when to make changes. To augment benefits that patients are receiving from their hearing instruments, our office has implemented an aural rehabilitation program. This program has helped our patients take ownership of their hearing problems, reduced their frustrations, and has increased the acceptance of their hearing instruments. Refer to Chapter 8 for details on rehabilitation programs.

CONCLUSIONS

Remember that hearing aid returns are typically a result of nonprofessional selling. Mistakes and omissions during the actual sales presentation, closing, fitting, and follow-up visits will sabotage successful hearing instrument fittings. You must examine each return for insight into future fittings. Change your process, educate your staff, provide training, or do whatever it takes to get patients in the door, purchase, and *keep* their hearing instruments. Make sure that you are selling professionally. Successful selling leads to a successful business and patients with better quality of life.

APPENDIX 6A

Patient Information Form

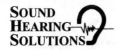

SOUND HEARING SOLUTIONS

| New Patient Information |

Name:	Age:

Address:

_____

_____
city   state   zip

Date of Birth:	Social Security No.:
Home Phone: ( )	Work Phone: ( )

Employer:

How did you hear about **SOUND HEARING SOLUTIONS?**

newspaper _____ radio _____ mail _____ friend (name, please) _____

doctor (name, please) _____ other _____

FOR OFFICE USE ONLY:

| Hearing Health History |

Description of Current Hearing Problems:	Primary Concern:
Medical History *ENT Physician:*_____ *Ear Surgery:* *Ear Infx/Drainage___ Tinnitus___ Vertigo___* *Earwax___* *Other Medical Issues:*	**Lifestyle** (work setting, clubs, hobbies, weekly activities, telephone, TV, automobile, etc.): **Special Problems** (vision, dexterity, memory, etc.):

HEARING AID HISTORY

Please read the following list. Check the appropriate areas in which you feel your current hearing aids need improvement.

Visibility _____   Telephone Use _____

Background Noise _____   Wind Noise _____

Feeling Stopped Up _____   Feedback (squealing) _____

Understanding in Quiet _____   Understanding in Noise _____

Soft Sounds Too Soft _____   Loud Sounds Too Loud _____

HEARING AID INFORMATION

Age of Hearing: _____

Where purchased: _____

OFFICE USE ONLY:

RIGHT		LEFT	
Brand	_____	Brand	_____
Model	_____	Model	_____
SN	_____	SN	_____
Battery Size	_____	Battery Size	_____

APPENDIX 6-B

The Listening Abilities Questionnaire

HEARING ABILITIES QUESTIONNAIRE

1. What is your hearing aid experience?

   ☐   I have a hearing device and use it regularly on the ___right ear ___left ear.

   ☐   I have a hearing device, but don't use it, or use it only occasionally.

   ☐   I tried a hearing device, but returned it for credit.

   ☐   I have inquired about hearing devices at another office(s), but did not purchase at that time.

   ☐   I have never used a hearing device.

2. Please rank the following from 1 to 4 in terms of their importance to you when purchasing a hearing device. (1 = most important and 4 = Least Important)

   ___ **Sound Quality & Clarity**   ___ **Durability/Reliability**   ___ **Cost**   ___ **Appearance**

3. What motivated you to come in today?

   _____

4. On a scale of 1-10, where do you feel that you are (psychologically, emotionally, financially, etc.) regarding doing something about your hearing loss? (Please circle one)

1	2	3	4	5	6	7	8	9	10
not motivated									very motivated

5. Please check the box which corresponds to your ability to hear in the situations listed and check how often you are in that situation.

Listening Situation	How well do you hear in this situation?			How often are you in this situation?		
	poor	fair	good	rarely	sometimes	often
Quiet Room (1 to 2 people)	☐	☐	☐	☐	☐	☐
Television	☐	☐	☐	☐	☐	☐
Music	☐	☐	☐	☐	☐	☐
Restaurants	☐	☐	☐	☐	☐	☐
Church	☐	☐	☐	☐	☐	☐
Meetings/Lectures	☐	☐	☐	☐	☐	☐
Work Place	☐	☐	☐	☐	☐	☐
Telephone Conversation	☐	☐	☐	☐	☐	☐
Car	☐	☐	☐	☐	☐	☐
Meal Times (at home)	☐	☐	☐	☐	☐	☐
Groups (4 to 6 people)	☐	☐	☐	☐	☐	☐
City Street	☐	☐	☐	☐	☐	☐
Large Social Gathering	☐	☐	☐	☐	☐	☐
Radio	☐	☐	☐	☐	☐	☐
Shopping	☐	☐	☐	☐	☐	☐

APPENDIX 6-C

Client Oriented Scale of Improvement (COSI)

COSI
The NAL Client Oriented Scale of Improvement

Date: 1. Needs Established   _____

              2. Outcome Assessed   _____

SPECIFIC NEEDS   **Indicate Order of Significance**

Degree of Change   "Because of the new hearing instruments, I now hear…"

Week: _____   Date: _____

☐   ☐   ☐   ☐   ☐   **Goal**

					Worse
					No Difference
					Slightly Better
					Better
					Much Better

Degree of Change   "Because of the new hearing instruments, I now hear…"

Week: _____   Date: _____

☐   ☐   ☐   ☐   ☐   **Goal**

					Worse
					No Difference
					Slightly Better
					Better
					Much Better

Degree of Change   "Because of the new hearing instruments, I now hear..."

Week: _____   Date: _____

☐   ☐   ☐   ☐   ☐   **Goal**

					Worse
					No Difference
					Slightly Better
					Better
					Much Better

Degree of Change   "Because of the new hearing instruments, I now hear..."

Week: _____   Date: _____

☐   ☐   ☐   ☐   ☐   **Goal**

					Worse
					No Difference
					Slightly Better
					Better
					Much Better

Degree of Change   "Because of the new hearing instruments, I now hear..."

Week: _____   Date: _____

☐   ☐   ☐   ☐   ☐   **Goal**

					Worse
					No Difference
					Slightly Better
					Better
					Much Better

Final Ability *(with hearing instrument)* "I can hear satisfactorily..."

Week: _____   Date: _____

☐   ☐   ☐   ☐   ☐   **Goal**

					Hardly Ever 10%
					Occasionally 25%
					Half the Time 50%
					Most of the Time 75%
					Almost Always 95%

APPENDIX 6-D

The Audibility Index

SOUND
HEARING
SOLUTIONS

NAME _____

DATE _____

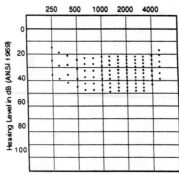

Audibility Index for Speech
(Mueller & Killion, 1990)

Frequency in Hz

Date		Condition	Ear	Status of Non-Test Ear		ST	Aud. Index
	△	Unaided		___ open ___ occluded			

Date		Make & Model	Ear	VC	Adjustments	ST	Aud. Index
	○						
	▢						
	●						
	■						

Comments:_____

_____

_____

_____

AUDIOLOGIST_____

6809 W. Northwest Hwy.   7777 Forest Ln., A-107   14902 Preston Rd., #407   1501 Redbud
Dallas, TX 75225   Dallas, TX 75230   Dallas, TX 75240   McKinney, TX 75069
(214) 691-5466   (972) 566-7643   (972) 702-8373   (972) 562-7270

APPENDIX 6-E

Hearing Aid Return Patient Profile

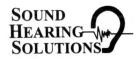

SOUND HEARING SOLUTIONS

HEARING AID RETURN
PATIENT PROFILE

Name:		M F	Date:
Hearing Aid Experience:	☐ Currently wears consistently ☐ Has HA's—doesn't wear ☐ Tried—returned for credit ☐ Inquired, but never bought ☐ Never tried HA's	**Age:** ☐ <50 ☐ 51-60 ☐ 61-70 ☐ 71-80 ☐ >81	**#1 Importance:** ☐ Sound Quality ☐ Durability ☐ Cost ☐ Appearance
Configuration of Hearing Loss:	☐ HF with normal lows ☐ HF with hearing loss in lows ☐ Flat ☐ Reverse Slope	**Referral Source:**	**Level of Motivation:**
Technology of Device (s) Returned:	☐ Digital ☐ Digitally Programmable ☐ Advanced ☐ Conventional	**Style of Device (s) Returned:** ☐ CIC ☐ ITC ☐ ITE ☐ BTE	**Was style appropriate for degree of HL? Y N**

TRIAL PERIOD HISTORY

Length of trial period: _____   Number of devices tried: _____

Number of follow-up visits: _____   Number of remakes: _____

Patient's reason for return: _____

_____

_____

_____

Specialist: _____   Office: _____

We have now reached the point in the process when the patient is ready to be fitted with his new hearing aids and finally listen to the new stimuli that are about to reach his brain. He is excited, and we are excited. He has been an active participant in the process and now he has reached another critical juncture. Before he leaves the specialist's office, he must have a thorough understanding of how the hearing aids work, how to begin wearing them, and what to expect they might do and not do for him. If the patient takes the hearing aids home without establishing realistic expectations or knowing how and when to utilize the instruments properly, the likelihood of failure is significantly increased. Thus, the professional is responsible for ensuring that these objectives are achieved before the patient takes the new devices out into the real world.

In Chapter 7, Elaine Mormer and Catherine Palmer present a systematic approach to hearing aid orientation. The complexity and sheer number of issues that need to be addressed at the fitting and orientation are such that clinicians cannot afford to forget certain topics or leave any "stones unturned." The approach you are about to learn is comprehensive, but is not without controversy. For example, many professionals believe that patients differ widely in their ability to adapt to new hearing aids; thus, they direct their experienced, and even some new patients, to begin wearing their hearing aids on a near full-time schedule as soon as possible. As the reader, it is your task to determine which approach best fits you and your patients' needs. Regardless of your view, I'm certain you will appreciate the fine attention to detail and systematic approach now presented.

7

A Systematic Program for Hearing Aid Orientation and Adjustment

■ **Elaine Mormer, M.A.** ■
■ **Catherine Palmer, Ph.D.** ■

This chapter contains a guide to the principles of hearing aid orientation and a systematic protocol by which these principles can be implemented. Hearing health care professionals readily agree that the style and content of the hearing instrument orientation has a significant impact on a patient's prognosis for amplification. The hearing aid orientation encompasses a number of components, all of which contribute to the patient's overall success using personal amplification. The format presented here is essentially a framework within which the specific needs of a patient can be addressed in an organized and thorough manner. Such a framework allows for individualized content addressing both the patient's distinct needs and the clinician's experience and style.

PRINCIPLES OF HEARING AID ORIENTATION

Consideration of Individual Needs

Patients require varying approaches to amplification orientation, depending on level of motivation, past experience, and personal learning style. Parents of young children require special attention, as they are usually the caretakers of the hearing instruments, without the direct experience of using the devices. Bingea, in Chapter 9, discusses this topic in detail. For parents, as for most new hearing instrument users, the initial introductory session can bring forth an emotional component of the hearing loss experience that may not have surfaced earlier. This element of the interaction may interfere with the patient's cognitive absorption of the materials presented. Thus, the need for printed materials reflecting all of the information presented cannot be overstated, as illustrated in the following dialogue.

Dispenser: Mrs. Kelly, I want to show you the parts of the hearing aid that you can see on the outside, so that you will understand a bit about how the hearing aid works. We'll start with the microphone here.

Mrs. Kelly (thinking to herself): Gee, these things really are much bigger than Florence's are. And I wonder why I don't need to have a remote control like she does. The girls at Bridge Club will be asking me about these things in my ears tonight.

Dispenser: And lastly, this is the part that fits into your ear canal.

Mrs. Kelly (thinking to herself): Gosh, I must really be getting old if I need to wear these all the time.

Motivational Factors

The source of a patient's motivation to use amplification will significantly affect the perceived success of the fitting. See Chapter 2 for details. For example, dispensers are rightfully hesitant to prescribe hearing aids for a reluctant elderly parent brought in by a frustrated adult son or daughter. This is not an uncommon scene in any dispenser's office, and most will agree that the source and level of motivation serve as a fairly solid indicator of the eventual outcome. In such scenarios it is important to determine whether the motivation to pursue amplification is generated from an internal (elderly mother really does want help with her hearing) versus an external source (adult son is tired of yelling into Mom's ear). This factor plays significantly into the content of the hearing aid orientation and adjustment counseling for patient and family members. Operation of higher level features such as T coil or alternative memories should not be introduced initially. Later, having recognized the benefit of this limited use of amplification, the patient can be instructed to use the instruments in a wider variety of situations while employing the breadth of technology features.

Prior Experience

First-time hearing aid users have different orientation requirements than those of experienced users. This is not meant to imply that orientation for experienced users is not necessary. Indeed, given the rapid pace with which hearing aid technology changes, the experienced user provides a particularly challenging orientation scenario. For example, the past user of a monaural linear type amplifier may bristle at the auditory sensation of a binaural wide dynamic range fitting, particularly if no volume control is included. The issues in this patient's orientation and adjustment plan need particular attention, with the focus diverting substantially from that of the first-time user. This scenario also requires a plan for adjusting to the addition of the second hearing aid, as well as an explanation of the instrument's ability to adjust the gain level automatically.

Learning Style

It is appropriate to inquire as to the patient's preferred learning mode. Some will readily acknowledge that they will not "read the manual." These patients do best with short checklists and repeated demonstration of operation and care. Other patients will look forward to getting home, where they will readily read through all of the manufacturer's literature, as well as any handouts from the dispenser. The astute clinician needs to be flexible in adapting to the individual patient's learning style.

The Hearing Aid as a Component of Aural Rehabilitation

The hearing instrument fitting is only one aspect of a patient's attempt to cope with the challenges of a confirmed hearing loss. Whether the hearing loss has been present for many years, or is of recent onset, the dispenser must consider a variety of issues with which each patient is dealing at an emotional level. Thus, *the successful hearing instrument orientation and adjustment must necessarily address issues of a personal and emotional nature.*

Areas of Personal Adjustment

The process of the hearing evaluation, medical clearance, and the decision to use amplification is cause for the successful hearing aid user to modify one's self-perception. This change need not be *negative* in the sense that the person with hearing loss thinks less of himself, but an altering of the self-image that now includes the need to use hearing instruments in the pursuit of the best quality of life. This self-perception seems to *evolve* rather than to *appear*, and the dispenser is wise to assess where in this emotional continuum the patient currently functions. Tools such as the Communication Profile for the Hearing Impaired (Demorest & Erdman, 1987) are helpful in assessing the patient's self-perception. Other indicators are the patient's willingness to seek outside help from books, the Internet, or self-help groups. It is certainly within the scope of the dispenser's role to guide the patient toward the end of the continuum where hearing loss and its impact are accepted and understood. This is the point at which the person with hearing loss will be best equipped to cope with his disability productively, increasing the chances for successful hearing aid use.

Another challenge facing the hearing instrument user involves adjustment to the fact that sound will no longer be heard naturally. The wearing of these instruments will indeed alter the user's life activities and routines, and family, co-workers, and/or friends will witness these alterations. For example, the new user may not anticipate difficulty wearing his hearing aids at the bowling alley or at trap shooting. The dispenser's guidance will be necessary not just in understanding how to fit the shell in the ear, but how to fit the instruments into existing daily routines.

Patient (a high school teacher): Do you think I'll be able to wear the aids to work after this week?

Dispenser: If you feel comfortable using them at home, in situations with some background noise, you should move on to using them at work.

Patient: The students in my class will notice that I have them, and I'm sure that they will expect me to hear their voices from the back of the room right away. I feel pretty timid about showing up with these in class.

Dispenser: It would probably be helpful if you take a few minutes before you start the class and explain that you just got these hearing aids. Show the students the hearing aids up close. Explain to them that it's important to you to hear each of the students when they speak in class. Does this sound like something you can realistically say to your students? You will still need to be fairly close to a student in order for the microphone to pick up his or her voice. Let's see how it goes and if we need to we can talk about some teacher/classroom listening strategies and technologies when you come back next time.

Trial Period as an Introductory Period

The first 30 days of hearing aid use have traditionally been referred to as the trial period. With stringent criteria for candidacy and fitting, one could argue that this period would be better labeled as the *Introductory* period, reflecting the ongoing adjustments (both electroacoustic and psychosocial) made as the dispenser and patient work together toward a successful hearing solution. This solution may consist of traditional hearing aids, assistive technology, communication strategies, or a combination of these. This philosophy is related to that described in the previous section, whereby amplification fitting is seen as only one part of the aural rehabilitation process. The dispenser, embracing the concept that she provides a service focused on maximizing communication ability, can offer alternatives when a particular amplification system does not meet the patient's needs. Additionally, some approaches to hearing aid fitting include tuning up (e.g., gradually increasing gain in certain frequency regions via reprogramming or potentiometer adjustments). If one follows this type of fitting strategy, *the true potential of the hearing aid may not be evident in the first 30 days of use.* (It should also be noted that some manufacturers are beginning to offer longer "trial" periods of up to 90 days.) Certainly, there will be patients who eventually reject any form of amplification. However, most who have been actively involved in the hearing rehabilitation process will have achieved at least some improvement in communication ability. *It is essential to counsel patients that hearing aid fitting is a process.* This process is still just *beginning* as the patient leaves the office with hearing aids for the first time.

Prognostic Indicators for Success

In our experience, several factors seem to be prognostic indicators for amplification success. The source and level of motivation, as mentioned previously, may be among the most significant factor. Also, it is critical to establish realistic expectations for the user, as discussed throughout this book. Likewise, the patient's general health and ability to participate in activities may have prognostic value, as well as guiding the type of technology chosen. For example, a frail elderly gentleman confined to a reclining wheelchair may make better use of a hard-wired assistive listening device than from custom fit hearing aids to engage in one-on-one conversation with his daughter.

The maintenance of interpersonal relationships nearly always depends on some form of productive communication. Thus, the involvement of family members or significant others is another critical factor in achieving a successful outcome. *At a minimum, patients should be asked to bring along a friend or family member to the initial hearing instrument orientation and to as many subsequent sessions as possible.* Whenever feasible, these significant others should be an important part of the orientation and adjustment procedures.

IMPLEMENTATION OF THE ORIENTATION SYSTEM

Why be Systematic?

Any clinical tasks or procedures are most effectively approached via an organized and systematic routine. Protocols are applied in all sorts of medical and therapeutic settings in an effort to address issues of consistency, thoroughness, and efficiency in the execution and documentation of clinical tasks. With a clearly laid out plan, and forms with which it will be implemented, the hearing aid dispenser avoids needing to think about what must be done, or what may have been left out. This is of particular importance in a multidispenser office, where patients trust that they will receive comparable services and attention regardless of the clinician in whose care they have been placed. Similarly, from a management perspective, a forms-based approach allows for standardization of operations, as well as the monitoring of interdispenser performance. Additionally, this systematic approach facilitates documentation of all clinical interactions and an organized approach to follow-up. These tasks are easily overlooked in the occasional frenzy of a busy practice.

Prefitting Considerations

As described earlier, several factors impact the hearing aid dispenser's choices in prescribing amplification solutions for an individual's listening needs. Thus, aspects of the orientation begin well in advance of the ordering or delivery of the instruments. For example, the establishment of realistic expectations can be conducted in a systematic manner using the Patient Expectation Worksheet to facilitate productive dispenser-patient interaction (see Appendix 7–A, Palmer and Mormer, 1997). This form was adapted from the COSI, Client Oriented Scale of Improvement (Dillon et al., 1991).

As can be seen on a partially completed version of the Patient Expectation Worksheet shown in Figure 7–1, the patient is asked to describe, in prioritized order, specific situations where communication difficulty interferes with a desired activity. The resulting situation, and the patient's perception of current success (hardly ever, occasionally, etc.), serve to further the dispenser's understanding of the patient's communication needs and goals. A "C" is entered on the form, based on the patient's description of *current* success, and then an "E" is recorded at the level of success at which the patient *expects* to function postfitting. These recorded levels serve as the starting point for the adjustment of expectations and/or dispenser decisions regarding the treatment approach. For example, the patient may express the desire to understand his wife's words as she repeatedly speaks to him from the top of the staircase while he watches television in the first floor family room of his spacious home. If the patient were left to expect that his new hearing aids will overcome this problem, he would likely be disappointed in their performance. The adjustment of this expectation might sound like the following dialogue.

Dispenser: Mr. Tucker, in this situation your hearing aids may not be able to compete with the sound from the television in order to hear your wife's distant voice. This is probably not a situation where hearing aids alone will offer a lot of help. There may be some other ways to address this difficulty. It would be helpful if your wife could come along to your next appointment here. At that point I'll be introducing you to your hearing aids, and it would be good for her to understand what to expect. If it is difficult for her to come down the stairs when she wants to talk to you maybe we could think about some type of signaling

Continued

Patient Expectation Worksheet

I am successful in this situation…

Goal (list in order of priority)	Hardly Ever	Occasionally	Half the Time	Most of the Time	Almost Always
1. Understand wife talking from top of stairs	C		√	E	
2. Understand speech during group visits after Moose Lodge meetings, in quiet		C			√ E
3. Hear sermon at small church, sitting in the front row		C		√	E
4. Converse with grandchildren on telephone	C			E	√(with T coil)
5.					

C = how the client functions currently (pre-treatment or with current technology/strategies)

E = how the client expects to function post intervention (HA, ALD, strategies, etc.)

√ = level of success that the audiologist realistically targets

A = how the client/family actually perceives level of success post fitting

Figure 7–1. Patient expectation and perception worksheet containing sample patient data.

system, or a wireless transmitter that would couple to your hearing aids.

Mr. Tucker: I think I may be able to convince my wife to come with me to my next appointment, but she's been talking to me from the top of the staircase for 43 years and that may be difficult to change! It sounds like you are telling me that with my hearing aids alone I may still hardly ever be successful hearing her from there.

Mr. Tucker's concern that his hearing aids will not improve his ability to hear his wife from the top of the stairs is a valid and important issue. The resolution of this issue will most certainly involve a change in behavior on the part of his wife, regardless of whether any other assistive technology is employed. Thus, the clinician moves on to the next prioritized situation, noting that the "top of the stairs" issue should be addressed when the wife is present at the hearing aid delivery/ orientation appointment.

Dispenser: That's right, and we should talk about this more when your wife is here with us. For now, let's move on to the next most important listening situation with which you feel that you need help.

Mr. Tucker: I'm missing a lot of the words that the guys are saying when we sit around talking after the weekly meeting at the Moose Lodge.

Dispenser (recording this on the form as the second situation described): Would you say that you are successful in this situation hardly ever, occasionally, half the time, most of the time, or what?

Mr. Tucker: I guess I would say occasionally, and it's usually pretty quiet in that room. A few of us usually stay late after everyone else leaves. I was figuring that with a hearing aid I should be able to understand the guys pretty much all the time.

Dispenser (marking a "C" in the "Occasionally" box, and an "E" in the "Almost Always" box): Well it seems to me that we should be able to improve your ability to understand in that situation to the "Almost Always" category.

Once completed, the Patient Expectation Worksheet results in a set of functional communication targets or goals that the dispenser and patient will hope to reach. In follow-up appointments that occur during the initial period of use, the dispenser refers to these goals and again questions the patient as to his current (aided) level of success. This format thus provides a measurement of outcome, as well as a tool by which to plan and modify treatment. A modified version of this instrument exists for pediatric patients (see Appendix 7–B, Palmer & Mormer, 1998) and is further discussed in Chapter 9. This tool is extremely useful in ensuring input and communication from parents, teachers, and other professionals involved with the child's education and/or (re)habilitation.

In addition to the above procedure, it is recommended that patients be provided with written materials aimed at introducing key concepts they will face as hearing aid users. There are a number of commercially produced patient education materials available on this topic. Hearing aid manufacturers often provide such materials to dispensers, who are wise to use them prior to the actual delivery. It is appropriate to give patients this information at the time that earmold impressions are taken. Recommended sources for this purpose include the Krames Communication brochure entitled "Hearing Aids," the Better Hearing Institute, Starkey's Aural Rehabilitation Review, or the Getting the Most Out of Your Hearing Aids video. Internet web sites and electronic bulletin boards additionally serve as rich resources with which to enhance patient education (see Appendix 7–C, Mormer & Palmer, 1998). The patient education handout, *Helpful Hearing Aid Expectations* (see Appendix 7–D) summarizes some of the important prefitting concepts that should be shared.

Delivery/Introduction

For purposes of this chapter it will be assumed that some form of verification (e.g., coupler or real ear measurements) of the hearing instruments is completed either prior to or during the patient's scheduled hearing aid delivery. The delivery appointment should begin with checking the physical and electroacoustic fit of the instruments. This should be done prior to any significant conversation relating to hearing aid introduction, because the actual wearing of the hearing aids should become part of any such discussion. The orientation should begin after the fitting has been appropriately verified and any necessary modifications have been made. It is critical at this point to include family members or significant others, whenever possible. For those patients who have significant difficulty understanding face-to-face conversation, an assistive listening device should be used during instruction. Alternatively, one hearing aid from a binaural set may be worn. A small sound level meter kept handy in the dispensing office will enable the dispenser to monitor the conversation level used. This is usually best kept at around 60 to 70 dB SPL to approximate normal conversation. The issue of conversational loudness often arises among family members, particularly spouses, and the use of the sound level meter can facilitate understanding (if not mediation) of such problems.

Two distinct areas of introduction need to be included at the initial delivery appointment. These include *operation* of the instruments and appropriate *use* of the instruments. The former relates mainly to the mechanical manipulation of the devices. The latter addresses the patient's need to incorporate these mechanical devices into existing family, school, work, and/or social activities. Both aspects are of equal importance in the orientation process.

Introducing Operation of the Instrument

The operation manual provided by the manufacturer is usually the best guide to follow in acquainting the patient with physical features of the instruments. Additional notes, including the dispenser's phone number, should be entered directly in the manufacturer's manual so that all the hearing aid-related information can be kept in one place in the patient's home. The introduction should begin with a tour of the physical landmarks on the hearing aid. A magnifying glass may be useful to have available with those patients who have visual impairment. The dispenser should follow the format of the manufacturer-provided manual, demonstrating operation of the volume control, battery insertion/removal, on/off/telephone switches, multiple memories, remote control, and so forth. Many patients need to be reminded that all of the information being presented is written in a book that will be taken home. In this manner, the patient is encouraged to listen actively and not to worry about memorizing information. The focus during this session should be directed at the patient's ability to operate the instrument. This would necessarily include the successful insertion and removal of the battery and earmold or shell, and manipulation of basic controls (as opposed to advanced features). Patients can be instructed to use the sticky tab from a new battery as a calendar marker so that battery life can be monitored.

Insertion of the earmold or shell is often an awkward maneuver for the first-time user. One useful approach is to begin by teaching the technique for removal of the shell. Once the patient has positioned his fingers to remove the instrument successfully, the position should be maintained for insertion. For behind-the-ear (BTE) hearing aids, this is sometimes best accomplished by beginning with the earmold alone, then adding the BTE case to the insertion scenario once the earmold has been mastered. It is also helpful to allow the patient some insertion and removal practice time, away from the dispenser's supervisory eyes. This can be done with the help of the significant other or with a mirror (provided that the reverse reflection is not confusing to the patient).

For some first-time users of hearing aids with multiple settings and/or advanced technologies (e.g., a combination BTE/FM hearing aid with auxiliary input and/or microphone), it may be necessary to limit the instruction to the operation of the main microphone setting. For these individuals, it is recommended that features be gradually integrated into the user's listening activities over a period of time.

Dispenser: Well, Mrs. Stevens, it looks like you won't have trouble putting in the earmolds, taking them out, and turning the hearing aids on and off.

Mrs. Stevens: Yes, but these other extra switches seem confusing to me!

Dispenser: I'd like you to take the hearing aids home today and use them for a week with the switch set only to "M" when you want them to be working.

Mrs. Stevens: Okay, but what about that other transmitter box you showed me was part of the hearing aid? When will I use that?

Dispenser: "That's the microphone and transmitter that you will ask the teacher at your Tai Chi class to wear so that you will be able to hear him better. But first it would be good for you to be using just the microphones that are built in to the hearing aids.

Certainly not every patient would require this gradual implementation of features. If the user understands and can demonstrate the ability to properly utilize the various options, the information can be presented and then reinforced at subsequent sessions. Thus, the dispenser needs to plan for the most appropriate introductory content on a case-by-case basis.

Instruction in cleaning and maintenance of the instruments should be given as described in the manufacturer's manual. It is advisable to teach patients to wipe off the canal portion of the earmold or hearing aid every time that the instrument is removed. Maintenance habits are formed early on in the adjustment process and should be monitored by the dispenser. Patients should be carefully instructed as to the use of wax picks and brushes, as overzealous use can be damaging to the vulnerable hearing aid receiver. In any case, before patients are sent home with the hearing aids, it is prudent to require that they demonstrate competency in insertion and removal of the batteries and earmolds/shells.

The Hearing Aid Operation Checklist As shown in Appendix 7–E, Palmer and Mormer (1997) provided a quick cheat sheet to which the dispenser can refer during this initial hearing aid teaching session. The checklist serves as a reminder, and as a means of documentation, that the basic components of instrument operation and care have been covered. Memories can be labeled for specified situations as they are introduced to the patient. Actual operation of the memory controls can be introduced at this time, if appropriate for the patient's technology skill and comfort level. The multimemory user should be instructed as to how to return to the main conversational memory at any time. This may be as simple as an on/off switch, removing and reinserting the battery, or pressing a button on the remote control. This method should be written in the user's manual, if it is not preprinted. This allows for a safety net and will help reduce frustration in the beginning of the introductory period. The Hearing Aid Operation form allows for customization of this information or other information reflecting the specific options or features included in a particular instrument.

Introducing Use of the Instruments

Having completed all of the items on the Hearing Aid Operation Checklist, the dispenser can now move on to introduce the use of the instruments. This format is used for both new and experienced users, requiring necessary modifications as per individual situations. *It is not safe to assume that experienced users can forego a detailed introduction to new instruments.* This is particularly true in the case of multi-memory instruments or those with updated features (e.g., direct audio input, remote control). The value of these higher priced instruments is only as good as the patient's ability to implement the advanced features. By the same token, an experienced monaural user being updated to a binaural fitting often will present the dispenser with a variety of adjustment challenges.

Discussion relative to instrument use should be conducted while the hearing aids are worn with volume controls set to a comfortable level. The sound level meter can be used to monitor that the 60 to 70 dB SPL level is maintained. The first topic covered relates to the patient's perception of hearing his own voice when the hearing aids are worn. The perception of one's own voice is often the first difficult hurdle of the hearing aid adjustment. Assuming that a long earmold canal (Killion, Wilbur, & Gudmundsen 1988), adequate venting, and appropriate electroacoustic modifications have been invoked, patients can be encouraged that they will eventually become accustomed to the sound of their own voice. The clinician can help to facilitate this adjustment with further explanation:

> **Dispenser:** Mr. McNamara, you probably haven't been aware that in addition to your difficulty hearing other people talking, you haven't been hearing your own voice the way you did before you had this hearing loss. As your hearing loss has gradually gotten worse, your perception of your own voice has gradually changed too. With your hearing aids we have suddenly changed the way that your voice sounds again, and you may really need some time to adjust to this change. Go ahead and count out loud from one to ten, then describe for me how your voice sounds to you. If necessary we can make some adjustments so that your voice sounds more comfortable. We do expect that your voice will sound *different*; however the difference should not be *intolerable* to you when you leave here today.

The patient who perennially complains of the *barrel effect*, or the sensation of talking *through my nose*, presents a challenge to the dispenser's expertise. These problems, usually associated with the occlusion effect, can be approached via venting, canal tubing, and/or electroacoustic modifications. However, any such modifications may compromise otherwise optimal sound quality, audibility, intelligibility, and feedback control. One way to diagnose the presence and/or degree of the occlusion effect is to insert the hearing aids or earmolds in the patient's ears in the proper position. Ask the patient to read or count aloud with the hearing aids turned off, then to describe the sound quality of his voice. In this manner the dispenser can begin to sort out the electroacoustic versus *plumbing* factors affecting the voice perception.

Assuming that the patient finds the aided sound of his own voice acceptable, the dispenser should then engage in some general conversation with, and among, the patient and family. Family members should be tactfully dissuaded from ill-conceived tests of the hearing aids' benefit:

Dispenser: Mr. Spencer, now that you have both hearing aids in and they feel comfortable for you, let's just talk for a bit to see how conversation sounds to you.

Mrs. Spencer (covering her mouth and whispering at 40 dB SPL as measured on the sound level meter): "Henry, what did we have for lunch today?

Mr. Spencer (straining to understand her question): Why Mildred, I heard you talking, but I couldn't seem to catch what you were saying just now.

Dispenser: It's important for both of you to understand that you will still need to use good communication strategies. For example, Mrs. Spencer, you should get your husband's attention before you speak to him. Also, make sure he can see your face when you're talking. The hearing aids will help him hear better, but his ability to understand speech clearly may still be limited when he can't see your face.

Mrs. Spencer: Oh, I see, but the real test will come when he tries to hear the preacher's sermon from our back row seats at church this Sunday.

Similarly, the patient fit monaurally to aid a unilateral or asymmetrical loss, should be dissuaded from *testing out* the aid by plugging up the unaided ear while listening to his wife. Patients should always be encouraged to use the residual hearing in both ears, as well as all available visual and contextual cues.

The concept of listening in competing background noise is then introduced. A controlled demonstration can be presented if the office does not allow for a realistically noisy experience. The dispenser should explain the inherent challenges of listening in noise. One way to demonstrate this is to turn on a multitalker babble tape, or other recorded noise, set at 65 dB SPL (creating a 5 dB signal-to-noise ratio at the patient's ear), angled from behind the patient's chair. The discussion can then be continued, focusing on Communication Strategies for the Hearing Impaired Listener (see Appendix 7–F) and Communication Tips for Talking with a Person with Hearing Loss (see Appendix 7–G).

For patients using multimemory hearing aids, this is a good time to demonstrate the use of the memories programmed for background noise. To demonstrate differences among programs, the introduction of background noise is essential. Without such noise, the listener will not perceive the benefit that the additional memory provides. Patients and significant others should be afforded ample opportunity to ask questions throughout the orientation session.

The Wearing Schedule: A Gradual Approach

The system presented here promotes a conservative introductory wearing schedule and precise directions for patients to follow during its implementation. (It should be noted that some audiologists may argue that not all patients require an approach that is this cautious.) The Wearing Schedule (see Figure 7–2, Palmer & Mormer, 1997) reflects an individualized plan that has been filled in for a particular patient. The Maximum In column refers to consecutive numbers of hours during which the hearing aids should be worn at a comfortable volume setting. Patients fit with binaural amplification are instructed that time "In" refers to binaural use. For the most part, it is *not* in the patient's interest to begin with one hearing aid and to add a second later. On the contrary, dispensing via a binaural attitude encourages patients to begin with two hearing aids (unless contraindicated) and later return one if necessary. The Minimum Out column refers to an unaided rest time. As noted on the example schedule shown, a number is assigned to each day that the hearing aid has been used (i.e., the day the hearing aid is dispensed = Day 1, the day after the hearing aid is dispensed = Day 2, etc.). Patients are instructed to keep the hearing aids in for not more than the number of consecutive hours equal to the days of use. For example, on Day 2, Mr. Spencer should not wear the hearing aids for more than 2 consecutive hours at a time. After each period of use, there should be a minimum of 1 hour of unaided time. Following this rest time, the hearing aids can be worn for the maximum consecutive number of hours allowed. This in/out sequence can be repeated throughout the patient's waking hours.

As seen in the farthest right column of the Wearing Schedule in Figure 7–2, patients can be directed to adjust gradually to using their hearing aids in increasingly challenging listening situations. Listening categories are assigned a letter value beginning with A equal to the least challenging to G equal to the most challenging. Two listening categories (H, I) are left open, to be customized for the patient. The dispenser assigns all categories to the day(s) deemed most appropriate based on anticipated level of difficulty for the individual. For exam-

Hearing Aid Wearing Schedule

Days of Use	Maximum In	Minimum Out	Maximum In	Listening Category
Day 1	1 hour	1 hour	1 hour	A+B
Day 2	2 hours	1 hour	2 hours	A+B
Day 3	3 hours	1 hour	3 hours	A+B
Day 4	4 hours	1 hour	4 hours	A+B+C
Day 5	5 hours	1 hour	5 hours	A+B+C
Day 6	6 hours	1 hour	6 hours	A+B+C+D
Day 7	7 hours	1 hour	7 hours	A+B+C+D
Day 8	8 hours	1 hour	8 hours	A+B+C+D+E
Day 9	9 hours	1 hour	9 hours	A+B+C+D+E+F+G

A. Inside your home, listening to quiet household sounds (e.g., water from faucet, toilet flushing, doorbell ringing, fan...).

B. Radio, television, quiet conversation with low background noise.

C. Quiet indoor work activities at home or office.

D. Quiet outdoor activities (e.g., gardening, walking, visiting in backyard).

E. Group conversation, dinner table discussion, entertaining visitors, driving car.

F. Theater, worship, classroom, other group listening.

G. Noisy work activities, back seat of car.

H. Other: _____.

I. Other: _____.

Figure 7–2.
Example hearing aid wearing schedule. (Reprinted with permission from Palmer, C., & Mormer, E., High Performance Hearing Solutions, Vol. 1: Counseling, Supplement to the *Hearing Review*, January 1997.)

ple, a patient who is timid about using new instruments may be advised to spend Day 1 wearing the hearing aids only for Category A activities. An active and outgoing retiree, who spends time gardening and visiting with neighbors, may do fine with Categories A, B, C, and D on Day 3.

As seen in the example schedule in Figure 7–2, patients are encouraged to begin hearing aid use in a quiet place at home, shortly after returning from the dispensing office. In fact, the authors' patients are instructed to remove their hearing aids and to wipe and store them properly before leaving the dispensing appointment. One of the reasons for this is to avoid the high noise levels present on the streets in our urban surrounding and in the noise that may accompany the bus ride or drive home. Patients are counseled that, once at home, the hearing aids should be inserted and a listening tour of the house should be made (sounds in Category A on the wearing schedule). Such sounds could include water running in the kitchen or bath, air conditioner, fan, doorbell ringing, toilet flushing, and so forth. After the first 1 hour rest time, the progression to radio, television, or quiet conversation can take place. The progression to more difficult listening situations is done in gradual steps, although the pace will vary depending on individual circumstances.

Experience has shown us that using this conservative approach to hearing aid adjustment serves to minimize any auditory and/or physical discomfort encountered by first-time users. Experienced users may similarly need time to adapt to the altered auditory image or physical fit introduced by new hearing instruments. There are data to suggest the need for a learning/adaptation period before the hearing aid user is using amplification and/or signal processing to its full advantage. (For a review of these findings see Palmer, Nelson, and Lindley, 1988.) For just this reason, we encourage all new patients, and many previous users, to follow the prescribed wearing schedule. A Wearing Schedule form where the Listening Category column has been left blank is provided (see Appendix 7–H) for the reader's use in customizing to individual philosophy and needs.

Special Considerations for Previous Users

As stated earlier, special challenges arise in the case of an experienced monaural user transitioning to binaural use. These listeners often require an extra amount of support as they adapt to the new binaural auditory sensation. In many ways it is appropriate to treat these patients as new listeners, directing them to wear the hearing aids only in a binaural manner, with a gradual increase in time and competing noise levels. Likewise, the patient who is rejecting high-frequency amplification because he was accustomed to previous aids that provided minimal or no gain above 3000 Hz may need additional planning. This adjustment period may include a gradual tuning up of the high-frequency response via a trimmer or programming over several weeks. Each previous user brings to the fitting past experiences that influence his impression of the new fitting. It is important to consider these past issues when planning for the fitting, orientation, and adjustment process.

Documenting the At-Home Experience

The most effective way to assess the patient's early experience with amplification is to encourage documentation during the first weeks of use. At the end of the introductory session, the Hearing Aid Commentary (see Figure 7–3, Palmer & Mormer, 1997) is provided to the patient for this purpose. The patient is asked to record notes on communication outcomes in the listening categories that are shown, using the variety of hearing aid configurations available for the fitting. This completed form is used to guide the follow-up visits. As seen in the sample Hearing Aid Commentary (Figure 7–3), blank spaces are available for the dispenser to customize to the individual's important auditory activities. In the example shown, the patient is a college student for whom classroom listening and fencing jousts present important communication challenges. The configurations of amplification should reflect realistic conditions of use for that patient. For example, if the patient has been instructed to switch to a directional microphone option while serving customers across the deli counter at work, this condition (directional microphone option ON) would be recorded as the configuration, while the listening category would be similarly described (serving customers over the deli counter). The sample Commentary reflects a patient using a new hearing aid with built-in FM receiver. As illustrated, the dispenser shades out the boxes that would not apply for a particular configuration (e.g., you would not use the FM setting to hear the telephone ring). Certainly not all patients will take the time to record in detail the outcomes of each experience. However, the follow-up appointments are considerably more productive when patients bring in even a few written comments, as opposed to general statements such as "this thing is too loud!" A blank Hearing Aid Commentary form is included in Appendix 7–I for the reader's use.

Before the patient leaves, a return appointment should be scheduled to occur in 1 to 2 weeks from the delivery date. Occasionally, a patient may appear likely to need some extra handholding so the follow-up appointment should be scheduled for some time in the next 3 to 4 days. In addition to the scheduled follow-up appointment, patients should be encouraged to call the dispenser's office *immediately* if questions or problems arise with the instruments. The dispenser's phone number should be clearly printed on the manufacturer's manual so that it is readily available to the patient. The approach here is to address problems while they are still small, avoiding a disastrous first week for the user (and possibly the dispenser).

Transferring Responsibility for Operation, Use, and Care

As the orientation session reaches its close, the dispenser and patient review and sign the Hearing Aid Consent form (see Appendix 7–J, Palmer & Mormer, 1997). This form serves as a checklist for the

Hearing Aid Commentary

Listening Category	Configuration 1	Configuration 2	Configuration 3	Configuration 4	Configuration 5
	No Hearing Aids	Hearing Aid Set to: mic	Hearing Aid Set to: FM	Hearing Aid Set to:FM+mic	
Quiet Conversation at home					
Conversation with background noise					
Dinner Table					
Watching TV					
Back Seat of Car					
Talking on Telephone					
Hearing Telephone Ring			XXXXXXXX XXXXXXX		
Classroom Listening					
Fencing					

Figure 7–3. Hearing aid commentary customized for patient use. (Reprinted with permission from Palmer, C., & Mormer, E., High Performance Hearing Solutions, Vol. 1: Counseling, Supplement to the *Hearing Review*, January 1997.)

dispenser to ensure that some basic information has been given to the patient. Requiring the patient to sign the form imparts to him some responsibility for implementing the instructions that were provided. It also serves as solid documentation that a thorough orientation was conducted. Additionally, patients can be given a handout summarizing the Americans with Disabilities Act (see Appendix 7–K, Palmer & Mormer, 1997). This information can serve to solidify the patient's understanding of the need for self-advocacy.

Follow-up Visits

When possible, it is a good idea to call new users within the first 2 to 3 days of the delivery. Patients are very responsive to this unexpected extra attention, and this call gives the dispenser a chance to head off any early developing problems. At this point, patients have usually come up with a new question or situation to discuss. It may become clear that they need to return sooner than the next scheduled visit (e.g., allergic to the earmold and "my ear canal is swollen but I was going to wait until my appointment with you in two weeks," or "my left hearing aid constantly whistles").

The Clinician Checklist for 1 to 2 Week Follow-Up Visit (see Appendix 7–L, Palmer & Mormer, 1997) guides the dispenser through the contents of this appointment. The items listed are addressed in terms of the need for further action or follow-up. For all the items listed on the checklist, space is provided for an action plan. This plan could vary from the need to add a wind hood, to modifying irritating contact points on an in-the-ear (ITE) shell. This organized list of follow-up needs is helpful to ensure that the necessary tasks are attended to in a timely manner. A check is placed in the right column when the action plan is successfully completed.

The Hearing Aid Commentary is referred to in an attempt to identify the strengths and weaknesses in the fitting. Comments on this sheet may lead the dispenser to recommend particular listening configurations or may point to unresolved problems that will require special assistive devices. As mentioned previously, for patients with telecoils and/or multiple memory hearing aids, demonstration and practice with these should be conducted at this visit (if not done earlier). It is critical for users (with and without telecoils) to practice listening on the telephone while at the dispenser's office. This is particularly important in order to determine the presence of feedback for devices without telecoils and to avoid the confusion that commonly arises from the misunderstanding of the telecoil feature when it is available. For users of multimemory technology, it is essential that they are both comfortable physically selecting each memory and that they understand which memory is to be used in a particular situation. The dispenser should provide a written map of how to select the memory for a particular situation. Phonak, Inc. includes a nice feature in their programmable software where the dispenser types in individualized memory descriptions. These are then printed out with the hearing aid information and can be given directly to the patient. Alternatively, the Hearing Aid Operation Checklist (see Appendix 7–E) contains spaces for designating situational uses of the memories.

Assessing Amplification Benefit

The Patient Expectation Worksheet (refer back to Figure 7–1) becomes an important vehicle for reviewing patient use and benefit at the follow-up visits. The original form is consulted, and the patient is again questioned as to his perceived level of success for the specified situations, with amplification in place:

Dispenser: Ms. Green, let's take a look at some of the situations you described as difficult for you, when you used your old (linear, single-channel, no telecoil, monaural) hearing aid. The technology that you are using now (wide dynamic range compression, multi-channel, pre-amp telecoil, binaural) should sound a bit different than what you were used to before. The first situation that you had described as a problem was hearing your co-workers in informal discussions in and around your cubicle at work. With your new hearing aids in, would you say that you are successful in this situation hardly ever, occasionally, half the time, most of the time, or almost always?

Ms. Green: I would say that I really am able to understand them almost always. But what I didn't know before was that my computer makes an intermittent whirring sound. My colleagues laughed at me when I asked if they too could hear their computer *thinking* when it is saving and processing data. I was shocked that they said they did! Also, I can definitely have a conversation with the guy in the cubicle behind me, but I also hear his newspaper pages being turned every morning as he reads the paper. In fact, I was hoping that you would adjust the hearing aids so that I wouldn't have to hear those sounds at all while I am at work.

Dispenser (marking an A in the Almost Always column): It sounds like you are describing the sound of the hard drive on your computer. How does the loudness of this sound compare to the conversation that goes on in the cubicle around you?

As illustrated in the above scenario, the solicitation of this situation-specific information gives the dispenser precise information as to where amplification adjustment and/or counseling efforts should be aimed. If the "A" mark falls short of the previously designated expectation, fine-tuning of the fitting or the expectation is in order. This patient's discussion may center on the fact that a successful hearing aid fitting brings back the entire world of sounds (including quiet environmental sounds that he may not have heard in many years). In essence, the hearing aid user must use his brain to tune out sounds just as the normal hearing individual does so long as the various sounds have a normal loudness relationship to one another. For instance, people talking to the individual should be perceived as louder than the computer hard drive humming. The Profile of Aided Loudness (Mueller & Palmer, 1998) may provide an important measure of the relative perceived loudness of soft, average, and loud sounds that the hearing aid wearer is encountering.

The sophisticated user who has mastered the operation and use of the hearing aids at this point may have no need to schedule further follow-up visits before a year has passed. Other patients may have return visits scheduled weekly until the hearing aids and/or batteries can be independently inserted and removed. Still others should come back after they have had a week or two of practice with previously unused advanced features. When adding new configurations or situations to the listener's repertoire, a new Hearing Aid Commentary form should be issued. Regardless of the return schedule, patients need to be notified as the expiration of the manufacturer's trial period approaches and then again as the warranty period nears its end. It is advisable to maintain some form of contact with users throughout the year to ensure continued satisfaction. Some dispensers use a customer satisfaction-type survey 90 days or more after purchase. Other options include battery clubs, newsletters, greeting cards, or promotional mailings, most of which can be somewhat automated once in place. The reader interested in assessing all aspects of his hearing aid delivery system is referred to the Practice Effectiveness Audit (Kotchkin, 1993). This is a checklist from point of contact to postfitting that allows for systematic evaluation of the dispenser's current attitudes, policies, and procedures.

SUMMARY

This chapter has presented a comprehensive system with which dispensers can guide patients through the orientation and adjustment period. It is based on the philosophy that a gradual approach to hearing aid acceptance yields a more satisfactory long-term outcome. Forms and handouts from this system can be implemented in their entirety or dispensers may choose to use parts from among them. If incorporated into the service delivery system, it is recommended that a packet of ready-to-use forms be inserted into each new patient file.

Tips for Successful Hearing Aid Orientation/Adjustment

1. Keep a sound level meter handy to monitor instructional conversation
2. Introduce background noise when demonstrating multimemory features
3. Insert shells/molds with *no* amplification on to assess occlusion effect
4. Do not assume that experienced users do not need thorough orientation
5. Have patient call a friend or relative from your office to practice using T coil
6. Instruct patient to take a listening tour of his/her house with the new aids
7. Instruct patient to use battery tabs as calendar markers of battery life
8. Maintain some form of periodic contact with patient through the first year

REFERENCES

Demorest, M., & Erdman, S. (1987). Development of the communication profile for the hearing impaired. *Journal of Speech and Hearing Disorders, 52,* 129–143.

Dillon, H., Koritschoner, E., Battaglia, J., Lovegrove, R., Ginis, J., Mavrias, G., Carnie, L., Ray, P., Forsythe, L., Towers, E., Goulisa, H., & Macaskill, F. (1991). Rehabilitation effectiveness: I. Assessing the needs of clients entering a national hearing rehabilitation program. *Australian Journal of Audiology, 13*(2), 55–65.

Killion, M., Wilber, L., & Gudmunsen, G. (1988). Zwislocki was right . . . A potential solution to the "hollow voice" problem (the amplified occlusion effect) with deeply seated earmolds. *Hearing Instruments, 39*(1), 14–18.

Kotchkin, S. (1993). Practice effectiveness audit questionnaire. Collaborative marketing campaign. Knowles Electronics, Inc., 1151 Maplewood Drive, Itasca, IL 60143 (703-250-5113).

Mormer, E., & Palmer, C. (1998). A guide to using the Internet: It could change the way you work. *The Hearing Journal, 15*(6), 29–31

Mueller, G., & Palmer, C. (1998). The Profile of Aided Loudness: A new "PAL" for '98. *Hearing Journal, 51*(1), 10–19.

Palmer, C., & Mormer, E. (1997). A systematic program for hearing aid orientation and adjustment. *The Hearing Review, High Performance Hearing Solutions Supplement, 1,* 45–52.

Palmer, C., & Mormer, E. (1998, February). Goals and expectations of the hearing aid fitting: Parent, child, educator. *Remediating Pediatric Hearing Loss Through Amplification: Taking Science into the Clinic.* An international symposium presented by the University of Pittsburgh, San Antonio, TX.

Palmer, C., Nelson, C., & Lindley, G. (1998). The functionally and physiologically plastic adult auditory system. *Journal of the Acoustical Society of America, 103,* 1705–1721.

APPENDIX 7–A

Patient Expectation and Perception Worksheet[1]

Patient Expectation Worksheet

I am successful in this situation…

Goal (list in order of priority)	Hardly Ever	Occasionally	Half the Time	Most of the Time	Almost Always
1.					
2.					
3.					
4.					
5.					

C = how the client functions currently (pre-treatment or with current technology/strategies)

E = how the client expects to function post intervention (HA, ALD, strategies, etc.)

√ = level of success that the audiologist realistically targets

A = how the client/family actually perceives level of success post fitting

[1]Reprinted with permission from Palmer, C., & Mormer, E., High Performance Hearing Solutions, Vol. 1: Counseling, Supplement to the *Hearing Review*, January 1997.

APPENDIX 7–B

Family Expectation Worksheet for Use with Pediatric Patients

Child is successful in this situation…

Goal (list in order of priority)	Hardly Ever	Occasionally	Half the Time	Most of the Time	Almost Always
1.					
2.					
3.					
4.					
5.					

C = how the child functions currently (pretreatment or with current technology/strategies)

E = how the child/family expects to function postintervention (HA, ALD, strategies, etc.)

√ = level of success that the audiologist realistically targets

A = how the child/family actually perceives level of success postintervention

APPENDIX 7–C

Internet Resources for People with Hearing Loss

Websites	URL
American Academy of Audiology, Consumer Resources	www.audiology.org/conshome.htm
American Academy of Otolaryngology: Assistive Communication Devices	www.drmongiardo.com/pated/~pe016.html
American Speech-Language-Hearing Association, Inc.	www.healthtouch.com/level1/leaflets/4860/aslha057.htm
ADA resources	www.public.iastate.edu/~sbilling/ada.html
The Say What Club	www.webcom.com/~houtx/swc2.htm
Travel Tips for Hearing Impaired People	www.netdoor.com/entinfo/herimaao.html
Association of Late Deafened Adults (ALDA) Inc.	www.alda.org

Discussion groups (Usenet Groups)

alt.support.hearing-loss
alt.support.tinnitus

List-serves

Beyond-Hearing	majordomo@acpub.duke.edu (subscribe BEYOND-HEARING First name, Last name)
Network for Overcoming Increased Silence Effectively (NOISE)	listserv@lists.acs.ohio-state.edu (subscribe NOISE First name, Last name)

APPENDIX 7–D

Helpful Hearing Aid Expectations Handout

1. I have just begun the *process* of adjusting to my hearing loss and the use of hearing aids.

2. My own voice may sound *different* when I am wearing my hearing aids.

3. I may have a new awareness of footsteps, door closings, newspaper rustling, and so forth.

4. Listening when background noise is present will still be challenging.

5. I may not know what questions to ask until I have used my new instruments for at least a few days.

6. My hearing aids are only part of the hearing rehabilitation services my dispenser supplies.

7. I will benefit most from amplification if I use speechreading and positive listening strategies along with it (e.g., I should not judge the effectiveness of hearing aids by asking people to cover their mouths when they speak).

For more information on what to expect from your hearing aids contact *insert your clinic name here, insert telephone number here, insert your address here.*

APPENDIX 7-E

Hearing Aid Operation Checklist[1]

1. ☐ Battery Insertion

2. ☐ On/Off function

3. ☐ Volume Control

4. ☐ Hearing Aid Removal

5. ☐ Hearing Aid Insertion

6. ☐ Telephone Coil

7. ☐ Remote /Multimemory Control

8. ☐ Cleaning

9. ☐ Memory 1/_____

10. ☐ Memory 2/_____

11. ☐ Memory 3/_____

12. ☐ Memory 4/_____

13. ☐ _____

14. ☐ _____

[1]Reprinted with permission from Palmer, C., & Mormer, E., High Performance Hearing Solutions, Vol. 1: Counseling, Supplement to the *Hearing Review,* January 1997.

APPENDIX 7–F

Communication Strategies for the Hearing-impaired Listener

1.   Learn to anticipate and understand the topic of conversation by using situational cues, contextual cues, and understanding of the logical sequence of events.

2.   Face the speaker directly and on the same level whenever possible. Sit across from and close to the speaker, with your better ear (if you have one) toward the speaker.

3.   In your home, reduce competing noises by turning off or lowering the volume of TVs, radios, stereo equipment, turning off running water, etc., for improved speech reception.

4.   Become familiar with the way different people express themselves: facial expression, vocabulary sentence structure, accent or dialect, etc.

5.   Maintain an active interest in people and events. Knowing about national and world affairs, as well as those of your community and friends, will help you to follow any discussion or conversation more readily.

6.   Utilize speechreading to the fullest!

    a.   Concentrate on the thought rather than individual words.

    b.   Do not interrupt the speaker until he/she has finished.

    c.   Observe expressions, gestures, and the face of the speaker.

7.   Remember that communication is a two-way exchange of information. Do not monopolize the conversation in an attempt to direct and control it.

8.   Remember to wear your hearing aids along with your glasses in order to benefit from the visual and auditory clues that become available.

For more information on how to improve upon and maximize communication if you are hard of hearing, contact *insert your clinic name here, insert your clinic telephone number here, insert your address here.*

APPENDIX 7–G

Communication Tips for Those Talking with a Person with Hearing Loss

1. Speak slowly, at a normal loudness level. Yelling distorts speech sounds.

2. Get the person's visual attention before you start speaking.

3. Do not exaggerate mouth movements to help with lipreading.

4. Make sure that your face and mouth are clearly visible.

5. Speak within a few feet of the listener.

6. Rephrase, rather than repeat missed words.

7. Clue the listener in as to the topic, or changes in the topic.

8. Do not eat, chew, or smoke while talking.

9. Move away from background noise, or turn off background TV, radio, running water.

10. Encourage the listener to let you know if he/she does not understand.

For more information on how to best communicate with your friend or family member with hearing loss, contact *insert your clinic name here, insert your clinic telephone number here, insert your address here.*

APPENDIX 7–H

Blank Hearing Aid Wearing Schedule

Days of Use	Maximum In	Minimum Out	Maximum In	Listening Category
Day 1	1 hour	1 hour	1 hour	
Day 2	2 hours	1 hour	2 hours	
Day 3	3 hours	1 hour	3 hours	
Day 4	4 hours	1 hour	4 hours	
Day 5	5 hours	1 hour	5 hours	
Day 6	6 hours	1 hour	6 hours	
Day 7	7 hours	1 hour	7 hours	
Day 8	8 hours	1 hour	8 hours	
Day 9	9 hours	1 hour	9 hours	

A. Inside your home, listening to quiet household sounds (e.g., water from faucet, toilet flushing, doorbell ringing, fan...).

B. Radio, television, quiet conversation with low background noise.

C. Quiet indoor work activities at home or office.

D. Quiet outdoor activities (e.g., gardening, walking, visiting in backyard).

E. Group conversation, dinner table discussion, entertaining visitors, driving car.

F. Theater, worship,classroom, other group listening.

G. Noisy work activities, back seat of car.

H. Other: _____.

I. Other: _____.

APPENDIX 7–I

Blank Hearing Aid Commentary Sheet

Listening Category	Configuration 1	Configuration 2	Configuration 3	Configuration 4	Configuration 5

APPENDIX 7–J

Hearing Aid Consent Form[1]

I have been provided with the following regarding my hearing aid fitting:

1. Information regarding the benefits of binaural vs. monaural hearing aid use.

2. Information on the use of the telephone coil or direct audio input with my hearing aids.

3. Information on special hearing aid circuitry or technology that may be appropriate for my hearing aid fitting.

4. Information on assistive listening and/or alerting devices available to maximize my communication ability and/or safety.

5. Information on the operation, maintenance, and use of my hearing aids.

6. Information regarding hearing aid insurance programs and the manufacturer's warranty of my instrument.

7. Information on the Americans with Disabilities Act (ADA) and my rights under this law.

8. Information regarding proper battery storage and the dangers of ingestion of hearing aid batteries.

_____   _____
Patient Signature   Date

_____   _____
Dispenser Signature   Date

[1]Reprinted with permission from Palmer, C., & Mormer, E., High Performance Hearing Solutions, Vol. 1: Counseling, Supplement to the *Hearing Review,* January 1997.

APPENDIX 7-K

Americans with Disability Act Information Handout[1]

THE AMERICANS WITH DISABILITIES ACT (ADA): The ADA was designed to ensure all people with disabilities access to goods, services, and facilities. This legislation provides protection in almost every aspect of society.

Title I: Employment
Title I of the ADA only applies to qualified individuals with disabilities, meaning only those individuals with or without reasonable accommodation, who can perform the essential functions of a particular employment position. This law prohibits employers from discrimination against a qualified individual with a disability in these areas: Job application procedures, hiring, discharge, compensation, advancement, and any other privileges of employment. These regulations not only include those individuals not already hired but also those individuals with disabilities who are currently employed. In some situations, **tax benefits** are available to employers when they comply with the ADA employment regulations.

Title II: State and Government
Title II of the ADA ensures that all people with disabilities can use all services, programs, and facilities of state and local government agencies. These agencies include schools, motor vehicle departments, police and fire departments; parks and recreation programs; jails and prisons; libraries, food stamp offices, welfare and social services; and public hospitals, clinics, and counseling centers. Under the ADA, a government cannot exclude a person with a disability from participating in a service; deny the benefits or services, programs or activities of the agency; or subject the person to discrimination by reason of the disability.

Title III: Public Accommodations
Under Title III of the ADA, persons with disabilities will have equal access to all public places such as theaters, restaurants, doctors' offices, bands, stores, and private schools. All of these facilities are required to provide auxiliary aids and services to ensure effective communication with deaf and hard of hearing individuals.

Auxiliary aids include such things as interpreters, telecommunication devices, written materials, assistive listening devices, and closed captioning. Also, public accommodations have to modify their policies to allow the use of guide or signal dogs. For existing facilities, the ADA requires that they remove any structural communication barriers. Any newly constructed building must be accessible to disabled individuals.

Title IV: Telecommunications
This regulation requires that all telephone companies provide local and long distance telecommunication relay service, 24 hours a day, from any location. Those individuals using this service may not be charged any more than a voice telephone user would be charged for the same call. Telephone companies also are required to publish information about their relay service. This includes their phone numbers in telephone books, billing inserts, and through directory assistance. Title IV also includes television. It mandates that all public service announcements that are produced or funded by the federal government include close captioning. After 1994, all new televisions with 13 inch screens or larger should have a computer chip built in that will decipher closed captioning.

[1]Reprinted with permission from Palmer, C. & Mormer, E., High Performance Hearing Solutions, Vol. 1: Counseling, Supplement to the *Hearing Review,* January 1997.

APPENDIX 7–L

Checklist for 1- to 2-Week Follow-up Visit[1]

ITEM	OUTCOME	ACTION PLAN	✓
Hearing Aid Commentary			
Hours Worn Per Day			
Able to Insert Aid			
Able to Remove Aid			
Cleaning & Maintenance			
Situations of Best Success			
Situations of Least Success			
Assistive Devices			
Aural Rehab Follow-Up			
Review Telephone Use			
Memory/Features Options			
Warranty Expiration			
Insurance Information			
Consent Form Signed			

✓ = Check off item if outcome is positive or when action plan is successfully completed.

_____   _____
Patient Signature   Date

_____   _____
Dispenser Signature   Date

[1]Reprinted with permission from Palmer, C., & Mormer, E., High Performance Hearing Solutions, Vol. 1: Counseling, Supplement to the *Hearing Review,* January 1997.

In the ideal world, all patients would now have reached "hearing nirvana." Orientation is complete, the patients have received a good education about hearing aids, and everything should be fine. In fact, the steps taken to this point may ensure that the patients keep their hearing aids and that you have avoided a return-for-credit situation. However, the reality is that our objective goes beyond getting the patients out the door and even through the 30-day "trial" period. Our goal is long-term satisfaction. This objective may be best achieved through serious audiologic rehabilitation. Again, remember that the hearing aids are only a portion of this process. In Chapter 8, Kathy Matonak places the role of hearing aids into perspective by offering a detailed description of audiologic rehabilitation. Many specialists are reluctant to carry the process this far because they fear that the amount of time and preparation required putting together an audiologic rehabilitation program would be cost and time prohibitive. These are legitimate concerns. A lot of thinking and preparation is required. In this chapter, much of this busy work and preparation has been completed for you. Various details of how to set up programs, and decisions regarding whether programs should be for groups or individuals, are discussed. In addition, a comprehensive set of references and materials found in the Appendix section will set responsible clinicians well on their way toward immediate implementation of this important next step in the process.

8

A Rehabilitation Program for Long-Term Success

■ Kathy Matonak, M.S. ■

The diagnostic audiologic evaluation, medical consultation, hearing instrument selection, fitting, and subjective and objective verification procedures have been completed. A great deal of time, talent, and financial resources has been expended. Expectations are high. What can we now do to ensure that the patient is achieving optimum communication competence and that the hearing instruments won't join the 17.9% of others that end up in a drawer or the 61% that are used half of the time (Kochkin, 1996)?

The answer is audiologic rehabilitation (AR). Until recently, this process was termed aural rehabilitation. The two differ in that aural rehabilitation traditionally consisted of training in lipreading, speechreading, and auditory skills. Audiologic rehabilitation, or rehabilitative audiology, on the other hand, consists of consideration and management of overall communication skills, psychosocial aspects of hearing loss, education of significant others, hearing aid orientation, emphasis on improving conversational and interactive skills, and use of assistive listening devices (Kricos & Lesner, 1996). The goal is long-term satisfaction, and participation in an AR program may be the most effective way to ensure that hearing aids will be worn (Montgomery, 1991). *It is essential not to assume that, although a patient may have an extended history of hearing loss and hearing aid usage, he would not benefit from rehabilitative audiology.*

Audiologic rehabilitation is rewarding for the recipient and provider. It can make a significant impact on our patients. Numerous researchers have reported that a decrease in self-perception of handicap can be shown for hearing aid use in combination with attendance in a counseling-based AR program versus receiving amplification alone (Abrams, Hnath-Chisolm, Guerreiras, & Ritterman, 1992; Kricos & Holmes, 1996; Weinstein, 1996).

The views expressed in this chapter represent an accumulation of the work of many writers and providers of audiologic rehabilitation. Among them are Ross, Abrahamson, Wayner, Kricos, Lesner, Palmer, Tye-Murray, Mormer, McCarthy, and Alpiner. In addition, the feedback and evaluation from present and past participants of AR programs are invaluable components in shaping existing and future programs.

GOALS OF AN AUDIOLOGIC REHABILITATION PROGRAM

Audiologic rehabilitation includes the combination of the use of hearing instruments, assistive listening devices, procedures, dissemination of information, interaction, and therapies that lessen the communicative and psychological consequences of hearing loss (Ross, 1997). *Hearing aids alone are not the total solution to the communication problems caused by hearing loss.* Despite the dramatic improvements in hearing aid technology in recent years, there has not been a similar increase in user satisfaction. The solution is not one strategy, one device, or one specific type of drill. A comprehensive, organized AR program could be designed to provide services to an individual, a group, or a combination of both.

Long-Term Goals

The long-term goals of an AR program are to:

■ optimize communication competence
■ provide long-term satisfaction
■ provide evaluation and management of the communicative and psychosocial implications of hearing loss

Short-Term Goals

Short-term goals vary depending on the topics covered in a particular session. Examples of short-term goals are to:

- encourage daily use of hearing aids
- include family members in the audiologic rehabilitation program
- reinforce the use of repair strategies
- identify auditory barriers that interfere with communicative competence
- identify nonauditory barriers that interfere with communicative competence
- encourage the use of coping strategies

Goal setting should be flexible. In general, the goals set for a group AR program will be similar to those set for an individual AR program. However, individual goals are more personal. They may include such personal goals as informing a boss and three co-workers that you have a hearing loss and are trying new hearing aids. Another personalized goal might be to join and attend local SHHH (Self-Help for the Hard of Hearing) group meetings.

WHY AUDIOLOGIC REHABILITATION PROGRAMS ARE OFTEN OMITTED

Audiologists are the logical professionals to provide AR to adults. Speech pathologists, educators of the deaf, and audiologists typically provide AR to children. There are three primary rationales used to justify why AR is *not* provided as a clinical service:

- Time (preparation for and presentation of the class)
- Limited training
- Lack of reimbursement

Time Restraints

Contrary to the belief that audiologic rehabilitation requires an abundance of time, one can argue that the communicative needs of many can be met simultaneously, thus actually saving time. Even with individual AR, the well-served patient requires less attention (time) in the long run. *Providing more effective education and realistic expectations to a patient will likely result in fewer return visits for the "perfect fit" and less time and income loss associated with returned hearing aids.*

Initially setting up a program admittedly does require time to decide on a curriculum, prepare materials, find a location, obtain necessary approvals, make appropriate purchases, and so forth. Preparation time before classes is needed, but decreases as the provider becomes more familiar and experienced. There are prepared materials and curriculum outlines ranging from a single 1-hour session (Montgomery, 1994) to multiple sessions (Kricos & Lesner, 1996; Palmer & Mormer, 1997; Wayner & Abrahamson, 1996) available that may minimize the initial preparation time required. Many are listed at the end of the chapter. Camera-ready materials are obtainable in the *Learning To Hear Again Program: An Audiologic Rehabilitation Curriculum Guide* (Wayner & Abrahamson, 1996). Samples of this program are provided later in this chapter. A one-session, 1-hour program called WATCH (Montgomery, 1994) that can be used as an introduction to AR consists of:

- **W** Watch the talker's mouth, not the eyes
- **A** Ask specific questions
- **T** Talk about your hearing loss
- **C** Change the situation
- **H** Healthcare knowledge

Training

Audiologic Rehabilitation

There are numerous workshops, books, videotapes, and articles on audiologic rehabilitation. The Academy of Dispensing Audiology (ADA), American Academy of Audiology (AAA), American Speech-Language-Hearing Association (ASHA), and Academy of Rehabilitative Audiology (ARA) provide sessions at conferences and journal articles. With the resurgence of AR, more educational materials are available, as evidenced by publications made available by leading publishing houses.

Counseling

Although it is acknowledged that counseling may be the single most important clinical service that hearing professionals provide, many audiology graduate programs do not provide formal coursework in it (Crandell, 1997). Consider taking a counseling course at a university or college if counseling is not your strength. These courses may be found in Education, Early Childhood Special Education, or Psychology departments, not just in Audiology programs. The different perspective provided by other diverse departments could be "enlightening."

Cultural Diversity

Training in Deaf Culture and Cultural Diversity may be obtained in community colleges and university classes. Books on Cultural Diversity, Deaf Culture, Deaf History, and American Sign Language are cited at the end of this chapter. Community Deaf Awareness activities are also available.

Reimbursement

Many audiologic rehabilitation programs have a fee associated with them. It can be a separate fee or part of the hearing aid purchase. Third-party payments are sometimes available. For example, if you perform pre- and posttherapy evaluations and complete all necessary paper-work, Medicare may reimburse for AR. Scholarships or fee waivers should be considered as motivating sources.

To be fair, however, it must be stated that, without funding, there are expenses associated with providing AR that need to be offset. Fortunately, there are secondary potential financial benefits that can be associated with successful programs:

■ Reduced return rate of hearing aids
■ Reduced return rate of assistive listening devices
■ Referrals of friends, co-workers, and family members
■ Reduction in number of troubleshooting visits
■ Free advertising provided by satisfied hearing aid users
■ Good community relations
■ Provision of comprehensive hearing health care as a marketing strategy
■ Hiring of audiologists by community colleges to provide AR
■ Grants for AR programs in the community from outside agencies, not-for-profit groups, foundations, or organizations

Further, the satisfaction of knowing that you have done the best job you can with all patients and that you have had a significant impact on their lives is rewarding in itself and helps minimize burn-out.

GENERAL ASPECTS OF AN AUDIOLOGIC REHABILITATION PROGRAM

Audiologic Rehabilitation Is a Process

A comprehensive AR program is an ongoing, evolving process. It is a process that includes client-centered counseling and the integration of many components to facilitate communication for long-term success. The process is dependent upon where the person is in the evaluative stage, the grieving stage, and the stage of behavioral change, as well as other considerations.

Process of Evaluation

The process of audiologic rehabilitation begins at the diagnostic evaluation. The information obtained through the history, the results of the evaluation, the discussion of the findings, and recommendations made are all essential to the eventual outcome.

The following is a list of outcome measures that can be used with patients and their families:

- Abbreviated Profile for Hearing Aid Benefit (APHAB)
- Hearing Handicap Inventory for the Elderly (HHIE)
- Hearing Handicap Inventory for the Elderly—Significant Other (HHIE-SO)
- Hearing Handicap Inventory for the Elderly—Screener (HHIE-S)
- Hearing Handicap Inventory for the Elderly—Significant Other Screener (HHIESO-S)
- Hearing Handicap Inventory for the Adult (HHIA)
- Hearing Handicap Inventory for the Adult—Significant Other (HHIA-SO)
- Hearing Handicap Inventory for the Adult—Screener (HHIA-S)
- Hearing Handicap Inventory for the Adult—Significant Other Screener (HHIASO-S)
- Client Oriented Scale of Improvement (COSI)

The screening versions of the Hearing Handicap Inventories (HHIA-S, HHIESO-S, HHIASO-S, HHIE-S [Appendix 8-A]) (Ventry & Weinstein, 1982) are completed during the audiologic evaluation appointment if hearing loss is present and communication difficulties are observed or expressed. If the score is 12 or greater, the patient is referred for hearing aids and an AR program. If the score is below 12, the patient is referred directly for AR, because it is not believed that these patients are ready to succeed with amplification at this time. At the completion of AR, however, many are ready to proceed with hearing aids and/or Assistive Listening Devices (ALD).

The process continues during the hearing aid evaluation/consultation appointment with self-assessment inventories that provide further information regarding handicap and disability and also provide outcome measures for benefit, expectations, and satisfaction. The Hearing Handicap Inventories can be used to assess handicap. Disability and hearing aid benefit can be analyzed using the APHAB (Abbreviated Profile for Hearing Aid Benefit) (Cox & Alexander, 1995) (Appendix 8-B). Expectations can be determined using National Acoustic Laboratories COSI (Client Oriented Scale of Improvement) (Dillon, James, & Ginis, 1997) shown in Appendix 8-C. Additional discussion of how these tools are used during the counseling process can be found in Chapter 7. The specialist must understand certain terminology in order to make the best use of these tools. The World Health Organization (Schow & Gatehouse, 1990) defined disorder, impairment, disability, and handicap as follows:

Disorder: a disease process or malformation of the system

Impairment: a loss or abnormality of psychological, physiological, or anatomical structure or function

Disability: a restriction or lack (resulting from an impairment) of ability to perform an activity in the manner or within the range considered normal for a human being

Handicap: a disadvantage for a given individual, resulting from an impairment or a disability, that limits or prevents the fulfillment of a role that is normal (depending on age, sex, social, and cultural factors) for that individual

Furthermore, satisfaction and benefit can be expressed as follows:

Satisfaction: a complex combination of benefit, communication needs, and personality traits

Benefit: advantages obtained from hearing aid use

Although hearing disabilities are the consequence of an individual's hearing impairment, it is the nonauditory effects of hearing impairment and hearing disability that combine to constitute a hearing handicap (Erdman, Work, & Montano, 1996). *An AR program can help prevent a hearing impairment from becoming a handicap.*

Grieving Process

The stages of grieving associated with death and dying (Kubler-Ross, 1969) also apply to individuals with hearing loss and their family members and are important considerations in the rehabilitative process. Position in a particular stage does not prevent a person from being included in a program; however it is important to be aware of the stage of grief the patient is in, and the possibility of relapse into a previous stage. The five stages that can be associated with hearing loss include:

1. *Denial.* The presence of hearing loss is denied (e.g., "I don't have a hearing loss. Young people don't know how to speak clearly.")
2. *Anger.* The presence of hearing loss and the communication difficulties associated with hearing loss can provoke an angry reaction (e.g., "Having a hearing loss is not fair. I'm a good person. Bad things shouldn't happen to good people.")
3. *Bargaining.* The person is trying to postpone the inevitable, often making "deals" of a spiritual nature (e.g., "If I become a better person, my hearing loss will go away.")
4. *Depression.* Loss of self esteem and social isolation (e.g., "I just haven't been myself lately. It's as though I'm in a fog.")
5. *Acceptance.* Neither angry nor depressed (e.g., "I'm sick and tired of missing out on what my grandchildren have to say, it's time for an ear trumpet.")

Process of Behavioral Change

A model of behavioral change based on the reduction of behaviors that contribute to health problems (Prochaska & Norcross, 1994) can be applied to the AR process. A change is not considered complete until termination is reached, and many individuals relapse into a previous stage. This model of behavior change is similar to the process that individuals with hearing loss go through during audiologic rehabilitation. It includes:

1. *Precontemplative.* No intention of changing; hasn't accepted that there's a problem (e.g., "I do just fine; no problems here.").
2. *Contemplative.* Aware of hearing loss; not yet committed to change, but collecting information (e.g., "I've had two different opinions from friends about hearing aids. I don't know who to believe. Eventually I've got to do something about this hearing loss.")
3. *Preparation.* Ready to take action (e.g., "I have an appointment next Tuesday to get my hearing tested.")
4. *Action.* A positive activity occurs (e.g., "I purchased two hearing aids.")
5. *Maintenance.* The benefit of the action is being realized (e.g., "The hearing aids are helping, but I want to get the most out of them for the long-term, so I signed up for a rehabilitation class.")

6. *Termination*. Accepted the action (e.g., "Buying the hearing aids and taking the AR class were the best things I've ever done for myself.")

Participation of Family, Friends, and Others

The inclusion of family members, friends, and significant others is essential to the process of improving communication. *It is important that communication partners understand that AR is a process, and their involvement in the process is integral in achieving a successful outcome.* After completing the hearing test, and before going over the results, the patient should be asked if there is someone in the waiting room he would like to have included. Hearing loss is a "family affair." The observation of the interaction between the patient and family, friends, or significant others provides an informal assessment of communication needs.

"She hears me when she wants to."
"If you'd only turn your hearing aid up."
"He talks too fast. If he'd just slow down I'm sure I could hear."
"I hear fine, I just don't understand what was said."

The patient is encouraged to include family, friends, or significant others in future evaluations, rehabilitation, or hearing aid related appointments. It is imperative that they understand the difficulties reduced auditory capabilities can present for the patient. It may be helpful to play a cassette of simulated hearing loss to help family members better understand what a high-frequency or a mild hearing loss is like. A better understanding of hearing loss promotes empathy. Something as simple as changing a behavior (i.e., it's not necessary to increase the volume of one's voice; it's better to slow down slightly the rate of speech) can make a world of difference. *The patient can also benefit sooner when multiple communication partners are involved in the program by learning about the impact that the hearing loss has on those around him.*

It is also useful to have a place to discuss the strategies and practice newly learned skills. It is critical to provide the opportunity to practice the skills, both in the rehabilitative setting and in the real world. Homework assignments may be given so that skills learned can be carried over to the home environment. Examples of assignments include:

- List helpful communication behaviors that occurred during the week
- Analyze the environment of the restaurant when dining out
- Identify barriers to effective communication
- Plan ahead for an activity to occur in the future
- Complete a communication profile and evaluation forms

AR should be organized so that it is fun. The patient, his family, friends, and significant others will enjoy it, and the reduction in communication difficulties and psychosocial effects of hearing loss will be appreciated.

Location and Facilities

The facility and its location are important considerations. Classes are provided in hospital settings; private physician's, audiologist's, hearing aid dispenser's, or speech pathologist's offices; speech and hearing departments at universities; community colleges; senior centers; convalescent homes; schools; churches; or at meetings. The location and facilities for group and individual programs can be similar; however, more options are available for individual sessions due to reduced room size requirements. The acoustics of the space, size of the training area, furniture, parking, temperature control, privacy, and lighting of the facility must be acceptable. The areas must be accessible (i.e., elevators, ramps, modified restrooms, etc.). They should have, or be close to, a coffee/hot water maker, refrigerator, microwave, restroom, and telephone. There should be ample audiovisual aids (e.g., television, VCR, projection screen, overhead projector, dri-erase boards, and large pads of paper on easels, etc.). A table and chair room set-up is preferred. Arranging chairs to face each other around a table so that patients can see each other, interact easily, and have a place for folders, beverage, and snack is helpful.

Respect for Cultural Diversity and Learning Style

Cultural differences and variations in learning styles must be acknowledged and respected.

Cultural Diversity

Cultural diversity is common and must be recognized. Providers of audiologic rehabilitation are encouraged to take classes in and read about Deaf Culture and cultural diversity.

Learning Styles

Selection of appropriate materials and activities based on whether the patient is a visual, auditory, or kinesthetic learner will facilitate learning and add to an atmosphere of comfort and trust. The differences in learning styles are reviewed at the beginning of the class; additionally, using combinations of visual, auditory, and kinesthetic methods for conveying information make classes more interesting.

Visual materials (e.g., handouts and overheads) should be kept simple and clear. Videotapes such as *Getting the Most out of Your Hearing Aids* and *Assistive Devices: Doorways to Independence* can be useful. Videotapes should be captioned, when available. Cassettes that simulate hearing loss such as those produced by the American Academy of Audiology and by Auditec have been employed; however, normal-hearing participants in the AR class should be cautioned that these tapes may not accurately simulate the cochlear and central auditory distortions experienced by many listeners who are hearing impaired. If this is not brought up, the devastating effect of certain hearing impairments may be underestimated. Ideally, the presenter will use assistive technology (e.g., sound field FM system, audio loop) when necessary to facilitate auditory reception during class. A personal amplifier should be offered to participants who do not have hearing aids and are experiencing difficulty hearing. Role-playing exercises may address the kinesthetic learner's needs.

Redundancy, repetition, and practice are important in learning any new information. Presenting information in varied ways and providing the opportunity to practice in both home and class environments will ensure success. People frequently will ask the facilitator questions that their audiologist and physician have previously addressed (i.e., about hearing and causes of hearing loss, etc.). Some of these individuals may not have heard or were too overwhelmed at the time the information was originally presented to them to comprehend and digest all the facts fully. Thus, the provider of AR should assume that all information is new. Refresher sessions should be provided periodically.

Individual Versus Group Audiologic Rehabilitation

Individual Audiologic Rehabilitation

Some patients live far away, are too fragile to be involved in a group setting, or have transportation or communication problems that preclude being part of an ongoing group. Individualized audiologic rehabilitation sessions can be designed to accommodate patients with special needs. Examples of patients who benefit from individual AR include the following:

■ A 20-year veteran realtor was having specific communication difficulties associated with his varied communication environments (e.g., automobiles, different telephone systems, house tours, numerous offices, etc.). He was recently embarrassed when confronted with his communication strategies of bluffing and monopolizing the conversation. His schedule precluded attendance at the prearranged group session time.

■ A businesswoman with significant hearing loss was experiencing stress and fatigue juggling home and work responsibilities as a single parent. Several areas of need were identified for her. The area that was causing her the most stress was that she worried that her children would eventually have hearing loss and she suspected hearing loss in her youngest child. She was new to the area and had not accessed medical services for her children yet. Her anxiety level and busy schedule precluded involvement in group sessions.

■ A well-known financial planner who lectured regularly was unable and unwilling to attend structured group audiologic rehabilitation classes. He was seriously considering early retirement because of the communication difficulties he was experiencing secondary to his hearing loss. It was clear that this gentleman required several individual sessions consisting of an informal needs assessment and development of a strategic plan that considered room layout, use of a remote microphone, and strategies to solicit questions.

■ One gentleman and his wife attended a group AR program, but after the second session it was recommended that, in addition to the group program, individual AR would be helpful. He recently experienced a sudden profound sensorineural hearing loss in his good ear, and had a severe-to-profound hearing loss in his other ear. He was not a good speechreader and did not know sign language. He very much wanted to be part of the group, but he had needs that were different from those of the rest of the group. To meet his need of belonging to the group, time was spent during the individual sessions preparing him for the group session so he could follow the class better. Additional visual materials (e.g., overheads, posters, and handouts) were prepared for his use.

■ An elderly man who was extremely talkative and rather hostile and pessimistic wanted to join an AR group. The facilitator felt that he would be disruptive to the group dynamics and individual therapy was offered as an alternative.

Individual sessions begin by having the patient review a typical day. Communication demands, auditory and nonauditory barriers to communication, and lifestyles issues are identified. Individualized strategies may be designed for attendance at religious services, participation in a legal case in court, involvement in organized sports, preparation for extensive travel abroad (e.g., communicating effectively with travel agents, renting automobiles, negotiating the airport, aircraft, gate changes, hotel reservations, etc.), and successful meeting attendance. *It is important to structure the individualized AR program so that early goals are ones that can be readily achieved, with more difficult to attain objectives coming later.* Because therapy is one to one, fewer sessions tend to be needed. Providers should be aware that *long-term individual AR is not usually cost effective.*

Group Audiologic Rehabilitation

Although less personal than individual AR, there is much to be said about the effects of a group. *Interchanges that occur in groups offer advantages and possibilities that cannot be met in individual follow-up appointments.* It may be quite comforting for patients to realize that they are not alone in their feelings and experiences. *Group members share and learn from each other, and encourage each other to acknowledge and take responsibility for their hearing loss.* They support each other. They occasionally become friends, and inquire about each other. An "our group" or "us" mentality is commonly developed. For certain individuals, a group program can be less threatening than an individual session. Homogeneity of the group may add to a nonthreatening atmosphere. It can also be more informative than individual sessions. The sharing of experiences and solutions is a dynamic process.

It is important to be able to practice the skills and solutions initially in a safe environment. For some, the group setting may supply the "safe" environment they need. They may recognize difficulties they weren't even aware of until expressed by a fellow group member. Some benefit from hearing solutions proposed by others. They "just hadn't thought of it that way." Some participants might be inspirational to other members. Participation in a group can help minimize the negative effects of hearing loss and permits significant others to be involved. Certain individuals, however, have a difficult time being assertive about their communication needs, and need to practice in private. For them, home practice with participation of significant others may be most appropriate.

Group AR is more cost-effective than individual AR and can be highly practical in a busy hospital-based program or private practice. Demonstrations of ALDs and hearing aids may translate into sales and effective listening habits. Group conversations can produce more realistic expectations among certain "unrealistic" participants and this could minimize the likelihood of hearing aid returns.

Instructional and Interactive Formats

Instructional Format

An instructional method of providing AR emphasizes the education of a patient by an "expert."

Interactive Format

The interactive format is one where the facilitator talks no more than 30% of the time. The members of the group discuss, share information, and problem solve. There is a high rate of family participation. Interactive methods are often rated higher by participants than instructional groups (Alpiner & McCarthy, 1993), but components of both can be beneficial.

The Role of the Facilitator

The provider is a facilitator of the dynamic process. The program encourages sharing and interaction. Because the group will ideally create a life of its own, the role of "expert" should be minimized, unless specific instruction to the group is called for. The facilitator prepares all materials, sets up the environment, oversees so that all members participate and have their needs met, and ensures that the discussion remains focused. All materials should be prepared in advance. Pens, pencils, name tags, handouts, videotapes, evaluation forms, markers for overheads, large pad of paper, dri-erase boards, and folders containing the group members' audiograms and suggested reading materials should be available. The folder should also include an empty envelope with the participant's name on it. Participants may request a copy of an article they saw on the bulletin board, a copy of a handout from last week that they lost, or an answer to a question they felt too shy to ask in front of the rest of the group. The requested information is retrieved during the week by the facilitator and returned in the envelope at the next session. Also inserted in the patients' folders can be a list of characteristics shared by successful AR participants (Wayner & Abrahamson, 1996).

This list might include:

■ consistent attendance and attention at sessions

- willingness to participate in class activities
- willingness to try new things
- willingness to share insights and experiences with others
- eagerness to learn from peers and interest in the success of others
- willingness to complete homework assignments and practice new skills outside of therapy
- willingness to examine long-standing communication behaviors
- willingness to include family and friends in the process of improving communication
- willingness to inform communication partners of the hearing loss and the associated needs
- willingness to be assertive in managing the hearing loss
- willingness to wear hearing aids routinely and use assistive technology whenever possible
- willingness to develop a sense of advocacy concerning the needs and rights of people with hearing impairment.

Hearing aids, accessories, and ALD's should be available for demonstrations. The function of all audiovisual equipment should be checked in advance. The facilitator may provide a snack and beverages.

Dealing with Disruptive Participants

Gatekeeping (i.e., assuring that no one member monopolizes the discussion) is essential to the process. A back-up plan for dealing with disruptive participants should be designed in advance. The disruptive person may be "monopolizing" the conversation, "putting down" others, not paying attention, or unwilling to participate in activities. It is important that the facilitator feels comfortable in redirecting and encouraging.

In addition, Wayner and Abrahamson (1996) suggest the facilitator needs to be able to:

- develop a trusting relationship with patients and family
- realize and convey to the patient that the hearing aid fitting is not the only step in AR
- determine when a hearing aid fitting alone is not sufficient to meet patients' communication needs
- be aware of the physical and mental changes that exist with hearing loss in older adults
- have the ability to modify evaluation and treatment procedures in ways that meet the needs of the individual patient

- develop the skills necessary to persuade administrators to invest resources of time and materials in rehabilitation services
- guide patients in the goal-setting process
- modify materials and oral presentation style to meet the needs of patients
- present information in a manner that is understandable and motivating to the patient
- modify interaction with patients to reflect awareness of cultural diversity in reactions to acquired hearing loss
- establish long-term relationships with patients
- conduct the intake interview in such a way that functional communication needs are addressed and initial rehabilitation goal formulation begins
- modify activities in groups to ensure that all participants are given practice items at appropriately challenging levels of difficulty

Traditional Versus Progressive Approaches in AR

Traditional Approach

The traditional approach includes the identification and evaluation of communication, lipreading, speechreading, and auditory training. The two techniques used in the traditional approach are termed *analytic* and *synthetic*. Analytic training includes structured drills focusing on the specific elements of speech in lipreading and auditory training. The synthetic approach focuses on the larger units of meaning, such as connected discourse, and environmental factors associated with listening. There are conflicting views regarding the effectiveness of these two approaches. It has been reported that analytic drills improved speech recognition in young adults (Walden, Erdman, Montgomery, Schwartz, & Prosek, 1981), but another study suggested that analytic drills were not helpful in improving a person's ability to understand speech in the presence of background noise (Kricos & Holmes, 1996). Instead, in the latter study, a synthetic approach emphasizing listening skills, coping strategies, nonverbal and situational cues, and modifications of environments to facilitate listening improved speech recognition and psychosocial functioning, especially in older adults. A logical conclusion from reviewing both schools of thought is that if one is to utilize a traditional approach, both analytic and synthetic components should be included.

Progressive Approach

The progressive approach can be seen as an extension of the traditional approach. The progressive approach includes identification and evaluation, client-centered counseling, and is goal-directed. The progressive approach encourages family involvement. It focuses on counseling, coping, and improved communication.

Other Considerations

Time Schedule

The times and days that classes are provided will be determined by many factors (i.e., availability of room, availability of facilitator, etc.). Midday and evening classes are recommended. Elderly patients and their spouses usually attend midday classes. Patients who are still in the workforce and their families generally prefer evening classes.

The number and length of sessions will be determined by the needs assessment. They may range from a single 1-hour meeting to as many as 24 sessions of individual therapy. Four to five 1- to 2-hour sessions is about average.

Number of Participants

The recommended group size is 6 to 12 members. Classes with more than 12 members may become more instructional than interactional. On the other hand, groups with fewer than 5 participants may not be able to develop or sustain the desired group dynamics to achieve maximum effectiveness. If this happens, it may be advisable to merge two small classes. Individual classes range in size from one to the number of family, friends, or significant others the patient would like to invite.

Advertising

Flyers describing the AR program with information regarding time, location, cost, and registration procedures should be available at audiologic evaluations and hearing aid consultations, when appropriate. These can also be distributed to otolaryngologists and certain general and family practice physicians, as well as your primary referral sources. Local newspaper and magazine coverage can be immensely helpful for promotional purposes.

Special Needs of Elderly Hearing-Impaired Patients

People are living longer. Presbycusis affects more and more seniors, and the degree of hearing loss gets worse with age. Central auditory processing difficulties may affect success with hearing aids. The auditory, mentioned above, and the nonauditory factors (Alpiner & McCarthy, 1993; Kricos & Lesner, 1996) listed below must be considered when planning presentations and providing AR services to the elderly.

Nonauditory Factors
Physical and Health Factors
- changes in vision
- changes in touch
- changes in pain sensitivity
- changes in health
- cutaneous changes

Psychological Factors
- learning
- memory
- motivation
- self esteem
- reaction time

Social Factors
- financial
- emotional
- mobility

Subject Matter for a Group Audiologic Rehabilitation Program

In the following section, a comprehensive list of subject matter for consideration is outlined. The specific topics included in any given program are a function of the needs of the participants, number and length of sessions, and the expertise of the facilitator. Therefore, the course content should be chosen and used as appropriate. Keep in mind that rehabilitative audiology is a dynamic process, constantly modified by changing needs, new ideas, and results of participants' evaluations.

It is assumed that the reader is familiar with the areas outlined. Topics that are somewhat uncommon are presented in greater detail. Topic-related handouts are available in the Appendix section of this chapter. The list of suggested readings at the end of the chapter should be consulted for further guidance.

1. Welcome and Introductions
   - Introduction of facilitator
   - Introduction of participants and taking attendance
   - Goals of the program
   - Goals of the session
   - General information

Structure, location, and times of class
Role of the facilitator
Restroom/break/telephone information
Availability of ALDs
Payment process
Review of folders—evaluation form, class materials,
  audiograms, homework materials, reference materials,
  applications for memberships, envelope, and facilita-
  tor's business card
- Ground rules
One person speaks at a time
No bluffing
Everyone gets a chance

2. Review of Audiologic Information
- Hearing and Hearing Loss
Symptoms of hearing loss (Appendix 8–D)
Anatomy and physiology of the ear
Causes of hearing loss (Appendix 8–E)
Types of hearing loss (Appendix 8–F)
Components of hearing loss
- Evaluation of hearing
Professionals associated with hearing, hearing loss, and
dispensing hearing aids
  Physician
  Audiologist
  Hearing Aid Dispenser
- Personal audiogram
- Configurations of hearing loss
- How hearing loss relates to speech perception
- Degrees of hearing loss—simulated hearing loss tape
- Common sounds audiogram (Appendix 8–G)
- Intensity of everyday sounds (Appendix 8–H)
- Conservation of hearing—distribute EAR earplugs
- Treatment of hearing loss
Medical
  surgical
  nonsurgical
Hearing instruments and assistive technology
Audiologic rehabilitation
  individual audiologic rehabilitation
  group audiologic rehabilitation
  new hearing aid user group

3. Psychosocial Aspects of Hearing Loss—12 Recurring Issues
    (Trychin, 1993)

- Depression. "This is not the life I thought I'd be living."
- Isolation. "I'd rather stay home."
- Anger. "If you'd only stop mumbling all the time."
- Exhaustion. "I'm exhausted after that meeting every time."
- Anxiety. "Needing hearing aids means I'm old."
- Insecurity. "What if I miss something."
- Despair. "This is hopeless."
- Negative self-image. "I'm not good at that anymore."
- Inability to relax. "I can't seem to slow down."
- Loss of group affiliation. "I gave up my theater tickets with the group."
- Paranoia. "He's out to get me fired."
- Loss of intimacy. "I miss being able to hear when my lover whispers to me."

4. Stages of Dealing with Hearing Loss (Kubler-Ross, 1969)
   - Denial
   - Anger
   - Bargaining
   - Depression
   - Acceptance

5. Implications of Hearing Loss
   - Communicative
   - Psychological
   - Educational
   - Vocational

6. Sources of Communication Difficulty and Strategies
   - External Sources
     background noise
     distance
     lighting
     seating arrangements
     distractions—auditory and visual
     beards
     accents
     rate of speech
     poor articulation
     acoustics of room
   - Internal Sources
     failing to understand the implications of the hearing loss
     hearing loss
     current communication strategies
       bluffing
       inattention

        dominating the conversation
      stress
      fatigue
      general health
      vision
      motivation to communicate
      personality

7. Communication Model
   - Speaker
     - rate of speech
     - how the message is delivered
     - loudness of speech
     - clarity of speech
       - articulation
       - accent
     - communicative behaviors
     - physical behaviors
   - Environment
     - distance
     - lighting
     - background noise
     - room acoustics
     - room ventilation
     - visual distractions
   - Listener
     - attention
     - fatigue
     - expectations
     - interest
     - knowledge
     - good use of hearing aids and/or ALDs
     - lipreading/speechreading skills
     - vision

8. Factors Influencing Understanding (Appendix 8-I)
9. Communication Strategies (Appendix 8-J)
   - Linguistic and situational cues
   - Reflective listening
   - Environmental management
   - Repair strategies
     - Repeat
     - Rephrase
     - Say or spell key word(s)
     - Summarize or simplify

Indicate the topic
Gesture
Confirmation
Question—specific and general
Write message—focus on key words
For numbers, say each digit individually
For letters, use alphabet, "B as in bat"
10. Auditory and Visual Strategies
   ■ Listening strategies (Appendix 8-K)
   ■ Communication guidelines (Appendix 8-L)
   ■ Rules for good communication (Appendix 8-M)
   ■ Speechreading (Appendix 8-N)
   ■ Lipreading
   ■ Tracking
      Repetition of continuous discourse
      Sender reads prepared text
      Receiver repeats text word for word
   ■ Effective listening (Appendix 8-O)
   ■ Active listening (Appendixes 8-P, 8-Q)
   ■ Assertive listening strategies (Appendix 8-R)
   ■ Auditory relearning
      Quiet . . . to presence of background noise
      One-on-one . . . to small group . . . to large group
      Inside home . . . to outside home
      Familiar sounds . . . to unfamiliar sounds
      Awareness . . . discrimination . . . identification . . .
         comprehension
11. Impact of Hearing Loss on Family
12. Hearing Aids
   ■ Styles of hearing instruments
      Body-borne
      Behind-the-ear (BTE)
      In-the-ear (ITE)
      Canal (ITC)
      Completely-in-the-canal (CIC)
   ■ Types of hearing instruments
      Conventional
      Hybrid (digitally programmable)
      Digital
   ■ Technological advances of hearing instruments
      Digital signal processing
      Directional and multiple microphones
      Multiple programs

Multiple channels
Tele-coils
Volume control
Direct audio input
■ Benefits and limitations of hearing instruments
Hearing instruments permit better use of residual hearing
Hearing instruments can improve day-to-day
communication
Hearing instruments cannot restore normal hearing
Hearing instruments cannot restore normal communica-
tion function
Central auditory processing difficulties can affect benefit
Hearing instruments require an adaptation period
The benefits of hearing aids are situation specific
■ Use and care of hearing instruments
■ Troubleshooting hearing instruments
■ Binaural advantages of hearing instruments
Localization of sound source
Squelch effect
Loudness summation
Elimination of head shadow effect
Consider trinaural fit (i.e., two hearing aids and one remote
microphone)
Remote transmitter/microphone placed close to the
sound source offers greater flexibility and enhanced
communication abilities
Consider BTE/FM
■ Steps to learning to use a hearing aid
■ Realistic expectations
12. Assistive Technology (Appendix 8-S) and Assistance Dogs
■ Interfering environmental factors
Background noise
Distance
Room acoustics
■ Considerations
Affordability
Effectiveness
Durability
Operability
Portability
Versatility
Mobility
Compatibility

Cosmetics
Previous experience
■ Types of ALDs
Auditory
Loudspeaker
Earphone
Direct-audio-input
Induction loop
Tactile
Fan
Vibrator
Dog
Visual
Captioning
Computer monitor
Fax
Lights
TTY
■ Alerting/signaling devices
Telephone
Doorbell
Alarm clock/watches
Smoke detector
Baby alarm
Personal pager
Siren indicator
Turn signal indicator
■ Large area assistive devices
Hardwired
Directly connected
Easiest
Least expensive
Infrared
Transmitter emits an invisible infrared light signal
Receiver picks up the signal
Must be in direct line-of-sight
FM—frequency modulation
Transmitter
Receiver
Radio signal
40 narrow-band frequencies
10 wide-band frequencies
Direct line-of-sight not needed

        Can be susceptible to interference

        Expensive

    Induction Loop

        Loop of wire is placed around a designated listening area

        Based on principle of electromagnetic induction

        Listener uses T-switch on hearing aid

        Dead spots can occur

■ Personal communication systems

    Telephone

        Amplifier

        Ringer

        TTY

        Local telephone company forms

    Television/stereo/radio

        Captioning

            Real

            Open

            Closed

    Theater

    House of worship

    Noisy environments

    Hearing dogs

    Other

        Amplified stethoscope

        Emergency care system

        TTY answering machine

13. Stress Management

  ■ Relaxation techniques

  ■ Coping strategies (Appendix 8-T)

    Anticipatory strategies

        Anticipate vocabulary

        Anticipate dialogue and sequence

        Anticipate and plan questions

        Anticipate and plan environmental concerns/
            modifications

        Consider how to be assertive

    Repair strategies. See #9 this section

  ■ Advocacy

    Legislation for people with hearing loss

        Americans with Disabilities Act

            Prohibits state and local governments and private businesses with more than 15 employees from discriminating based on hearing impairment

Established the dual party relay system for calls within and between the states

Employment

State and local governments

Public accommodation

Telecommunications

The Rehabilitation Act of 1973: Section 504

Prohibits federal agencies or business with federal government contracts of >$10,000 or recipients of federal financial assistance from discriminating based on hearing impairment

Public School Education PL94-142

Least restrictive environment for educational purposes of school-age individuals

Television Decoder Circuitry Act

By July 1, 1993, all TVs with screens 13" or larger must have built-in closed-captioning

Telecommunications Accessibility Enhancement Act 1988

Provides for telephone access to federal agencies

Provides access to all federal offices

Hearing Aid Compatibility Act of 1998

All telephones manufactured for sale in the United States after August, 1989 must be hearing aid compatible. The same for cordless telephones by 1990

13. Organizations
   - Self-help for hard of hearing (SHHH)
      Nonprofit educational organization
      Bimonthly journal: *SHHH Hearing Loss*
      Annual convention
      State associations, chapters, and groups
      Application for membership, national
   - American Tinnitus Association (ATA)
      Nonprofit organization
      Education-advocacy-research-support
      Annual convention
      Quarterly journal: *Tinnitus Today*
      Application for membership

14. Cochlear Implants
   - Surgically implanted devices for adults and children with severe-to-profound hearing loss
   - Electrodes stimulate the nerve of hearing when electrical signals are coded and received

- A microphone picks up sounds and sends them to a sound processor where they are amplified, filtered, and digitized
- Many assistive listening devices can be coupled to cochlear implants with special cords

Outcome Measures and Audiologic Rehabilitation Programs

Outcome measurement tools specifically designed for audiologic rehabilitation programs and the adjustment to hearing loss are needed. A short, easy to administer questionnaire that addresses all aspects of AR for patients and their families is needed. Testimonials and anecdotal reports are readily available.

The measurement tools listed in this chapter as well as a number of others provide useful information on hearing aid benefit, user satisfaction and expectation, handicap, and disability. The information obtained from these instruments can help target individuals in need of an individual or group AR program, and identify specific needs. Documentation for hospital administration, accrediting bodies, consumers, or third party payers can be achieved by using the self-assessment inventories.

SUMMARY AND CONCLUSIONS

This chapter has highlighted, outlined, and organized several aspects that are important for individual and/or group AR. The information provided here should be helpful to professionals interested in developing AR programs for their patients. Specific handouts, provided in the Appendixes, offer additional details of the issues listed in the outline. The main points of this chapter are summarized as follows:

1. To ensure long-term satisfaction and communicative competence, include audiologic rehabilitation in the clinical services you provide.
2. To ensure success, view audiologic rehabilitation as a process that begins at the diagnostic audiologic evaluation, not after the hearing aid fitting.
3. Patient-centered, family-oriented programming is critical to success.
4. Individual sessions can be a substitute or complement to the recommended group audiologic rehabilitation program.
5. Discuss and consider assistive technology with every patient who is hearing impaired.
6. Be sensitive to the cultural diversity and learning styles of others.
7. Prepared curriculum materials are available.

8. An AR program can help prevent a hearing impairment from becoming a handicap.
9. Providing AR can be rewarding to both the recipient and facilitator.

REFERENCES

Abrams, H., Hnath-Chisolm, T., Guerreiros, S., & Ritterman, S. (1992). The effects of intervention strategy on self perception of hearing handicap. *Ear and Hearing, 13*(5), 371–377.

Alpiner, J. A., & McCarthy, P. A. (1993). *Rehabilitative audiology: Children and adults* (2nd ed.). Baltimore: Williams & Wilkins.

Cox, R., & Alexander, C. (1995). The Abbreviated Profile of Hearing Aid Benefit. *Ear and Hearing, 16*(2), 176–186.

Crandell, C. (1977). An update on counseling instruction within audiology programs. *Journal of the Academy of Rehabilitative Audiology, 30,* 77–86.

Dillon, H., James, A., & Ginis, J. (1997). Client oriented scale of improvement (COSI) and its relationship to several other measures of benefit and satisfaction provided by hearing aids. *Journal of the American Academy of Audiology, 8,* 27–43.

Erdman, S. A., Work, D. J., & Montano, J. J. (1996). Implications of service delivery models in Audiology. *Journal of Aural Rehabilitation Academy, 27,* 45–60.

Kochkin, S. (1996). Customer satisfaction and subjective benefit with high performance hearing instruments. *Hearing Review, 3*(12), 16–26.

Kricos, P. B., & Holmes, A. (1996). Efficacy of audiologic rehabilitation for older adults. *Journal of the American Academy of Audiology, 7,* 219–229.

Kricos, P. B., & Lesner, S. A. (Eds.). (1996). *Hearing care for the older adult: Audiologic rehabilitation.* Boston: Butterworth-Heinemann.

Kubler-Ross, E. (1969). *On death and dying.* New York: Macmillan.

Montgomery, A. (1991). Aural rehabilitation: Review and preview. In G. A. Studebacker, F. H. Bess, & L. B. Beck (Eds.), *The Vanderbilt hearing aid report II.* (pp. 223–231). Parkton, MD: York Press.

Montgomery, A. (1994). WATCH: A practical approach to brief audiologic rehabilitation. *Hearing Journal, 47*(10), 10, 53–55.

Palmer, C., & Mormer, E. (1997). A systematic program for hearing instrument orientation and adjustment. *Hearing Review 1* (Suppl.), 45–52.

Prochaska, J. O., & Norcross, J. C. (1994). *Systems of psychotherapy: A transtheoretical approach* (3rd ed.). Pacific Grove, CA: Brooks/Cole.

Ross, M. (1997). A retrospective look at the future of aural rehabilitation. *Journal of the Academy of Rehabilitative Audiology, 30,* 11–28.

Schow, R., & Gatehouse, S. (1990). Fundamental issues in self-assessment of hearing. *Ear and Hearing, 11*(5 Suppl.), 6S–16S.

Trychin, S. (1993). *Communication issues as they relate to hearing loss.* Washington, DC: Gallaudet University Press.

Ventry, I., & Weinstein, B. (1982). The hearing handicap inventory for the elderly: A new tool. *Ear and Hearing, 3,* 128–134.

Ventry, I., & Weinstein, B. (1983). Identification of elderly people with hearing problems. *Asha, 25,* 37–47.

Walden, B., Erdman, S., Montgomery, A., Schwartz, D., & Prosek, R. (1981). Some effects of training of speech recognition by hearing-impaired adults. *Journal of Speech and Hearing Research, 24,* 207–216.

Wayner, D. S., & Abrahamson, J. E. (1996). *Learning to hear again: An audiologic rehabilitation curriculum guide.* Austin, TX: Hear Again Publishing.

Weinstein, B. (1986). Validity of a screening protocol for identifying elderly people with hearing problems. *Asha, 28,* 41–45.

Weinstein, B. (1996). Treatment efficacy: Hearing aids in the treatment of hearing loss in adults. *Journal of Speech and Hearing Research, 39*(5, Suppl.), S37–S45.

RESOURCES

Suggested Readings

Abrahamson, J. (1996). Effective and relevant programming. In P. Kricos & S. Lesner (Eds.), *Hearing care for the older adult: Audiologic rehabilitation* (pp. 75–111). Boston: Butterworth-Heinemann.

Abrahamson, J. (1997). Patient education and peer interaction facilitate hearing aid adjustment. *Hearing Review, 1*(Suppl.), 19–22.

Alpiner, J. (1973) Aural rehabilitation in the aged client. *Audecibel, 22,* 102–104.

Baker, C., & Battison, R. (1980). *Sign language and the Deaf community.* Silver Spring, MD: National Association of the Deaf.

Binnie, C., & Hessian, C. (1990). A four week communication skillbuilding program. *Academy of Dispensing Audiologists Feedback, 2*(1), 37–41.

Cox, R. (1997). Administration and application of the APHAB. *The Hearing Journal, 50*(4), 32–48.

Erber, N. (1993). *Communication and adult hearing loss.* Abbotsford, Australia: Clavis.

Gagne, J. P., & Tye-Murray, N. (Eds.). (1994). Research in audiological rehabilitation: Current trends and future directions [Monograph]. *Journal of the Academy of Rehabilitative Audiology, 4*(Suppl. 27).

Gannon, J. (1981). *Deaf heritage: A narrative history of Deaf Americans.* Silver Spring, MD: National Association of the Deaf.

Garstecki, D. (1996). Older adults: Hearing handicap and hearing aid management. *American Journal of Audiology, 5,* 25–34.

Garstecki, D., & Erler, S. (1997). Counseling older adult hearing instrument candidates. *Hearing Review 1*(Suppl.), 14–18.

Geier, K. (Ed.). (1996). *Handbook of self-assessment and verification measures of communication performance.* Columbia, SC: Academy of Dispensing Audiology.

Kochkin, S. (1993a). MarketTrak III: Higher hearing aid sales don't signal better market penetration. *Hearing Journal, 46*(7), 47–54.

Kochkin, S., (1993b). MarkeTrak III: Key factors in determining customer satisfaction. *Hearing Journal, 46*(8), 39–44.

Kochkin, S. (1993c). Practice effectiveness audit questionnaire: Collaborative marketing campaign. Itasca, IL: Knowles Electronics, Inc..

Kochkin, S. (1996). MarketTrak IV: Ten years of trends in the hearing aid market—has anything changed? *Hearing Journal, 49*(1), 23–34.

Kricos, P. B. (1997). Audiologic rehabilitation for the elderly: A collaborative approach. *The Hearing Journal, 50*(2), 10–19.

Lesner, S. (1992). Hearing disorders management in patients with presbycusis. *Hearing Instruments, 45,* 11–22.

McCarthy, P. (1996). Hearing aid fitting and audiologic rehabilitation: A complementary relationship. *American Journal of Audiology, 5*(2), 24–28.

McCarthy, P., Montgomery, A., & Mueller, H. (1990). Decision making in rehabilitative Audiology. *Journal of the American Academy of Audiology, 1,* 23–30.

Mueller, H. G. (1997). Outcome measures: The truth about your hearing aid fittings. *The Hearing Journal, 50*(4), 21–31.

Myers, I. (1962). Manual for the Myers Briggs Type Indicator. Palo Alto, CA: Consulting Psychologist Press, Inc.

National Center for Health Statistics. (1994). Prevalence and characteristics of persons with hearing trouble: United States 1990–1991 (Series 10, #188). Washington, DC: U.S. Department for Health Statistics.

National Center for Law and Deafness. (1992). *Legal rights: The guide for deaf and hard of hearing people.* Washington, DC: Gallaudet University Press.

Northern, J. L., & Sanders, D. A. (1972). Philosophical considerations in aural rehabilitation. In J. Katz (Ed.), *Handbook of clinical audiology* (pp. 685–694). Baltimore: Williams and Wilkins.

Padden, C., & Humphries, T. (1988). *Deaf in America: Voices from a culture.* Cambridge, MA: Harvard University Press.

Palmer, C. (1995). Deprivation, acclimatization, adaptation: What do they mean for your hearing aid fittings? *Hearing Journal, 47*(5), 10, 41–45.

Palmer, C., Butts, S., Lindley, G., & Snyder, S. (1996). *Time out! I didn't hear you.* Pittsburgh, PA: Sports Support Syndicate, Inc.

Ross, M. (1997). Reflections on binaural hearing aid fittings. *The Hearing Journal, 50*(40) 10–18.

Schow, R. L. & Nerbonne, M. A. (1989). *Introduction to aural rehabilitation* (2nd ed.). Austin, TX: Pro-Ed.

Singer, J., Healey, J., & Preece, J. (1997). Hearing instruments: A psychological and behavioral perspective. *Hearing Review, 1*(Suppl.), 23–27.

Smedley, T., & Schow, R. (1990). Frustrations with hearing aid use: Candid observations from the elderly. *Hearing Journal, 43,* 21–27.

Trychin, S. (1982). *Did I do that?* Bethesda, MD: SHHH Publications.

Trychin, S. (1994, July/August). Getting beyond hearing loss: A guide for families. *SHHH Journal.*

Trychin, S. & Boone, M. (1987). *Communication rules for hard of hearing people.* Bethesda, MD: SHHH Publications.

Tye-Murray, N. (1991). Repair strategy usage by hearing impaired adults and changes following communication therapy. *Journal of Speech and Hearing Research, 34*(4), 921–928.

Tye-Murray, N. (1998). *Foundations of aural rehabilitation.* San Diego: Singular Publishing Group, Inc.

Tye-Murray, N., Purdy, S., & Woodworth, G. (1992). Reported use of communication strategies by SHHH members: Client, talker and situation variables. *Journal of Speech and Hearing Research, 35,* 705–717.

Wilcox, S. (Ed.). (1989). *American Deaf culture: An anthology.* Burtonville, MD: Linstok Press.

Wilkinson, D. (1995). Counseling: Every patient is different. *Hearing Journal, 48*(7), 63–67.

Williot, J. F. (1996). Physiological plasticity in the auditory system and its possible relevance to hearing aid use, deprivation effects, and acclimatization. *Ear and Hearing, 17,* 665–775.

Wood, C., & Miettinen, I. (1988). Why you should have a hearing therapist. *Journal of Laryngology and Otology, 102,* 142–143.

Videotapes

Assistive Devices: Doorways to Independence. (1991). Cynthia Compton, Gallaudet University, 800 Florida Avenue, NE, Washington, DC 20002. Available through the Academy of Dispensing Audiologists (800) 454-8629. Manual and tape.

Getting the Most out of Your Hearing Aids. (1994), C. Everett Koop, M.D., CDR Communications, 9310-B Old Keene Mill Road, Burke, VA 22015-4204. (800) 557-HEAR.

Tinnitus. American Tinnitus Association P.O. Box 5, Portland, OR 97207 (503) 248-9985

Audio Cassettes

Simulation of Hearing Loss. Auditec of St. Louis
Say What? American Academy of Audiology (see Organizations)

Curriculums

Learning To Hear Again: An Audiologic Rehabilitation Curriculum Guide. Donna Wayner and Judy Abrahamson, 1200 Madison Avenue, Austin, TX 78757. (512) 479-9300 Website: http://www.HearAgainPublishing.com

Organizations

Self Help for Hard of Hearing People, Inc. (SHHH). 7800 Wisconsin Avenue, Bethesda, MD 20814. (301) 657-2248 (Voice), (301) 657-2249 (TTY)

American Tinnitus Association (ATA), P.O. Box 5 Portland, OR 97207. (503) 248-9985

American Academy of Audiology (AAA), P.O. Box 3676 Washington, DC 20007. (703) 610-9022 (Voice), (800) 222-2336 (Toll free), (703) 610-9005 (Fax), Website: http://www.audiology.org

Academy of Dispensing Audiologists (ADA), 3008 Mullwood Avenue, Columbia, SC 29205. (803) 252-5646 (Voice), (803) 765-0860 (Fax), e-mail: info@audiologist.org Website: http://www.hear4u.com

Academy of Rehabilitative Audiology (ARA), P.O. Box 26532, Minneapolis, MN 55426. (612) 920-0196 (Voice), (612) 920-6098 (Fax)

American Speech-Language-Hearing Association (ASHA), 10801 Rockville Pike, Rockville, MD 20852. (301) 897-5700

APPENDIX 8–A

Hearing Handicap Inventory for The Elderly—Screener

INSTRUCTIONS: The purpose of this questionnaire is to identify the problems your hearing loss may be causing you. Circle Yes, Sometimes, or No, for each question. **DO NOT SKIP A QUESTION IF YOU AVOID A SITUATION BECAUSE OF A HEARING PROBLEM.**

E-1   Does your hearing problem cause you to feel embarrassed when meeting new people?   Yes Sometimes No

E-2   Does a hearing problem cause you to feel frustrated when talking to members of your family?   Yes Sometimes No

S-1   Do you have difficulty hearing when someone speaks in a whisper?   Yes Sometimes No

E-3   Do you feel handicapped by a hearing problem?   Yes Sometimes No

S-2   Does a hearing problem cause you difficulty when visiting friends, relatives, or neighbors?   Yes Sometimes No

S-3   Does a hearing problem cause you to attend religious services less often than you would like?   Yes Sometimes No

E-4   Does a hearing problem cause you to have arguments with family members?   Yes Sometimes No

S-4   Does a hearing problem cause you difficulty when listening to the TV or radio?   Yes Sometimes No

E-5   Do you feel that any difficulty with your hearing limits or hampers your personal or social life?   Yes Sometimes No

S-5   Does a hearing problem cause you difficulty when at a restaurant with relatives or friends?   Yes Sometimes No

Score E: Score S: Score T:

Source: From Weinstein, B. (1986) Validity of a screening protocol for identifying elderly people with hearing problems. *Asha, 28* 41–45. Reprinted with permission.

APPENDIX 8–B

Abbreviated Profile of Hearing Aid Benefit

INSTRUCTIONS: Please circle the answers that come closest to your everyday experience. Notice that each choice includes a percentage. You can use this to help you decide on your answer. For example, if a statement is true about 75% of the time, circle C for that item. If you have not experienced the situation we describe, try to think of a similar situation that you have been in and respond for that situation. If you have no idea, leave that item blank.

A Always (99%)
B Almost Always (87%)
C Generally (75%)
D Half-the-time (50%)
E Occasionally (25%)
F Seldom (12%)
G Never (1%)

	Without My Hearing Aid	With My Hearing Aid
1. When I am in a crowded grocery store, talking with the cashier, I can follow the conversation.	A B C D E F G	A B C D E F G
2. I miss a lot of information when I'm listening to a lecture.	A B C D E F G	A B C D E F G
3. Unexpected sounds, like a smoke detector or alarm bell, are uncomfortable.	A B C D E F G	A B C D E F G
4. I have difficulty hearing a conversation when I'm with one of my family at home.	A B C D E F G	A B C D E F G
5. I have trouble understanding dialogue in a movie or at the theater.	A B C D E F G	A B C D E F G

6. When I am listening to the news on the car radio, and family members are talking, I have trouble hearing the news.   A B C D E F G A B C D E F G

7. When I am at the dinner table with several people, and am trying to have a conversation with one person, understanding speech is difficult.   A B C D E F G A B C D E F G

8. Traffic noises are too loud.   A B C D E F G A B C D E F G

9. When I am talking with someone across a large empty room, I understand the words.   A B C D E F G A B C D E F G

10. When I am in a small office, interviewing or answering questions, I have difficulty following the conversation.   A B C D E F G A B C D E F G

11. When I am in a theater watching a movie or play, and the people around me are whispering and rustling paper wrappers, I can still make out the dialogue.   A B C D E F G A B C D E F G

12. When I am having a quiet conversation with a friend, I have difficulty understanding.   A B C D E F G A B C D E F G

13. The sounds of running water, such as a toilet or shower, are uncomfortably loud.   A B C D E F G A B C D E F G

14. When a speaker is addressing a small group, and everyone is listening quietly, I have to strain to understand.   A B C D E F G A B C D E F G

15. When I'm in a quiet conversation with my doctor in an examination room, it is hard to follow the conversation.

A B C D E F G   A B C D E F G

16. I can understand conversations even when several people are talking.

A B C D E F G   A B C D E F G

17. The sounds of construction work are uncomfortably loud.

A B C D E F G   A B C D E F G

18. It's hard for me to understand what is being said at lectures or church services.

A B C D E F G   A B C D E F G

19. I can communicate with others when we are in a crowd.

A B C D E F G   A B C D E F G

20. The sound of a fire engine siren close by is so loud that I need to cover my ears.

A B C D E F G   A B C D E F G

21. I can follow the words of a sermon when listening to a religious service.

A B C D E F G   A B C D E F G

22. The sound of screeching tires is uncomfortably loud.

A B C D E F G   A B C D E F G

23. I have to ask people to repeat themselves in one on one conversation in a quiet room.

A B C D E F G   A B C D E F G

24. I have trouble understanding others when an air conditioner or fan is on.

A B C D E F G   A B C D E F G

Source: Reprinted with permission from Cox, R., & Alexander, C. (1995). The abbreviated profile of hearing aid benefit. *Ear and Hearing, 16*(2), 176–186.

APPENDIX 8–C

Client Oriented Scale of Improvement

Name: _____

Audiologist: _____ Category. New _____

Date: 1. Needs Established _____ Return _____

      2. Outcome Assessed _____

SPECIFIC NEEDS

Indicate Order of Significance

Degree of Change						CATEGORY	Final Ability (with hearing aid) Person can hear				
Worse	No difference	Slightly Better	Better	Much Better			10% Hardly Ever	25% Occasionally	50% Half the Time	75% Most of Time	95% Almost Always

Categories

1. Conversation with 1 or 2 in quiet
2. Conversation with 1 or 2 in noise
3. Conversation with group in quiet
4. Conversation with group in noise
5. Television / Radio @ normal volume
6. Familiar speaker on phone
7. Unfamiliar speaker on phone
8. Hearing phone ring from another room
9. Hear front door bell or knock
10. Hear traffic
11. Increased social contact
12. Feel embarrassed or stupid
13. Feeling left out
14. Feeling upset or angry
15. Church or meeting
16. Other

Source: Dillon, H., James, A., & Ginis, J. (1997). Client oriented scale of improvement (COSI) and its relationship to several other measures of benefit and satisfaction provided by hearing aids. *Journal of the American Academy of Audiology, 8,* 27–43. Reprinted with permission.

APPENDIX 8–D

Symptoms of Hearing Loss

- Asking for repeats
- Accusing others of mumbling
- Having difficulty hearing speech from a distance
- Having difficulty hearing in the presence of background noise
- Preferring the radio or television louder than what is necessary for others in the family
- Having difficulty understanding what is said on the telephone
- Having difficulty hearing young children's voices
- Having difficulty hearing women's voices
- Having difficulty hearing softly spoken speech
- Speaking louder than is needed
- Being told by a family member, friend, co-worker, or significant other that they suspect you have hearing loss
- Cupping your ear for improved hearing
- Having difficulty localizing the source of sound
- Favoring one ear over the other
- Straining to hear
- Tiring easily after attending a lecture, movie, or meeting
- Experiencing a change in your speech
- Finding it easier when the speaker's face is visible to you
- Missing more of the conversation than usual
- Experiencing difficulty hearing in group settings
- Using "what" and "huh" more often
- Avoiding groups
- Guessing more often
- Suffering from eye strain
- Having difficulty hearing soft sounds
- Finding that loud sounds are annoying

APPENDIX 8–E

Possible Causes of Hearing Loss

- Genetic Predisposition
- Head Trauma
- History of Ear Infections
- Excessive Ear Wax
- Noise Exposure
- Heart Disease
- Viral Infection(s)
- Ototoxic Medications
- Ménière's Disease
- Foreign Body in Ear Canal
- Acoustic Tumors
- Thyroid Problems
- Diabetes
- Perforated Ear Drum
- Growth in Ear Canal
- Growth in Middle Ear Space
- Birth Defect
- Presbycusis

APPENDIX 8-F

Types of Hearing Loss

Conductive

- Problem in the outer or middle ear
- Often temporary
- Can be treated medically and/or surgically
- Obstruction of the sound pathway from the outer or middle ear to the inner ear

Sensorineural

- Problem in the inner ear or auditory nerve, sound is not being transmitted properly
- Often permanent
- Often not treated medically and/or surgically
- Remediated most often with hearing aids, assistive listening devices, and audiologic rehabilitation

Mixed

- Has a conductive and sensorineural component

APPENDIX 8–G

Audiogram of Familiar Sounds

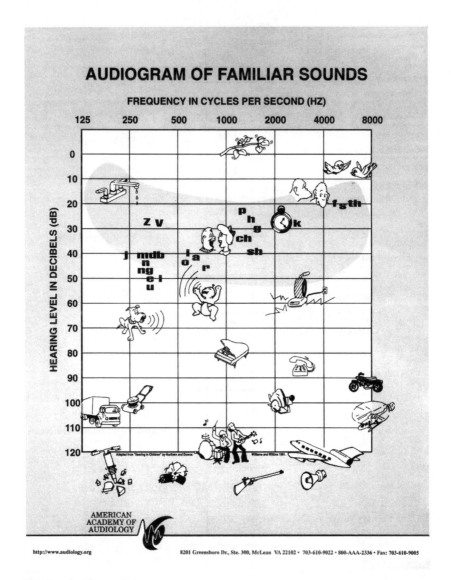

Reprinted with permission.

APPENDIX 8–H

Relative Loudness Levels of Common Sounds

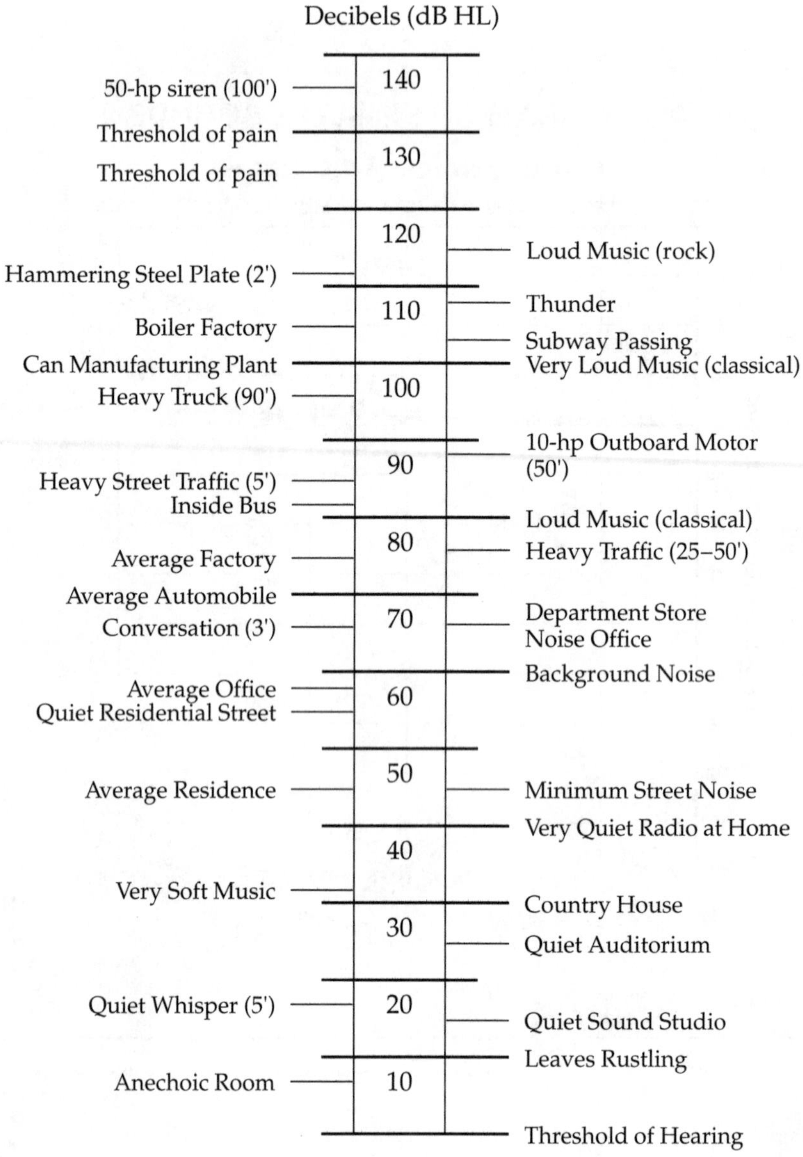

Decibels (dB HL)

Left side	dB	Right side
50-hp siren (100')	140	
Threshold of pain		
Threshold of pain	130	
	120	Loud Music (rock)
Hammering Steel Plate (2')		
	110	Thunder
Boiler Factory		Subway Passing
Can Manufacturing Plant		Very Loud Music (classical)
Heavy Truck (90')	100	
	90	10-hp Outboard Motor (50')
Heavy Street Traffic (5')		
Inside Bus		
	80	Loud Music (classical)
Average Factory		Heavy Traffic (25–50')
Average Automobile		
Conversation (3')	70	Department Store Noise Office
Average Office	60	Background Noise
Quiet Residential Street		
	50	Minimum Street Noise
Average Residence		Very Quiet Radio at Home
	40	
Very Soft Music		Country House
	30	Quiet Auditorium
Quiet Whisper (5')	20	
		Quiet Sound Studio
		Leaves Rustling
Anechoic Room	10	
		Threshold of Hearing

Source: From Wayner, D., & Abrahamson, J. (1996). *Learning to Hear Again.* Austin, TX: Hear Again Publishing. Reprinted with permission.

APPENDIX 8–I

Factors that Influence Understanding

Listener
- Level of hearing loss
- Type of hearing loss
- Use of hearing aids and/or assistive devices
- Attention level
- Motivation to hear
- Expectations
- Emotional state
- Fatigue
- Distracting thoughts
- Speechreading skills
- Tinnitus
- Tension level
- Manual communication

Speaker
- Voice intensity
- Voice projection
- Rate of speech
- Clarity of speech
- Facial expression
- Body language
- Foreign accent
- Facing listener
- Monotonous tone
- Beard or mustache
- Emotionality
- Mannerisms
- Objects at mouth
- Interest in message
- Relationship to listener

Environment
- Background noise
- Lighting conditions
- Room acoustics
- Distance from source of sound
- Assistive devices
- Distractions
- Use of visual aids
- Readability of visual aids
- Interfering objects
- Angle of vision

Source: From Wayner, D., & Abrahamson, J. (1996). *Learing to Hear Again.* Austin, TX: Hear Again Publishing. Reprinted with permission.

APPENDIX 8–J

Communication Strategies

■ Make it a habit to watch the speaker even if listening is not difficult. It is good to get in the habit of paying attention.

■ Don't interrupt the speaker before he/she finishes a sentence. You may not understand the beginning, but may catch the end.

■ When you are aware that you missed something that was said, ask for it to be repeated.

■ Summarize what you did hear so that your communication partner knows what to fill in.

■ Learn the topic being discussed. When you know what a person is talking about, it is easier to follow the conversation.

■ Learn to look for ideas rather than isolated words.

■ Keep alert for "key words" in sentences in order to follow ideas.

■ Use the clues from the situation to help get meanings. The idea is often spelled out by the actual situation. You may be able to anticipate words or phrases that will probably be used.

■ Don't be afraid to guess using situational and contextual clues.

■ Keep informed of your friends' interests. If you and your friends have favorite topics, this limited content makes understanding easier.

■ Stay aware of current events. When you know something about a topic, you can more readily recognize key words, names, etc. It will be helpful to read the daily newspaper and to be aware of the programs many people may watch, even if you don't watch TV.

■ Ask family members to keep you informed about things that are happening in your community and neighborhood and about events in the lives of people you know.

■ Keep your sense of humor.

Source: From Wayner, D., & Abrahamson, J. (1996). *Learning to Hear Again.* Austin, TX: Hear Again Publishing. Reprinted with permission.

APPENDIX 8–K

Listening Strategies

■ Ask the speaker to speak in a good light and face the listener.

■ Ask the speaker to speak clearly and naturally but not to shout or exaggerate articulatory movements.

■ Ask the speaker to repeat the message if it is not understood or to say it another way

■ When entering a group in the middle of a conversation, ask one person to sum up the gist of the conversation.

■ If someone is speaking at a distance, move closer.

■ If a speaker turns his or her head away, ask the speaker to face the listener.

■ If conversation is occurring in the presence of noise, try to move yourself and the speaker to a quieter area.

■ When in a communication situation requiring exact information such as directions or schedules, it is well to obtain the crucial information in writing.

■ Ask the speaker not to speak while eating, smoking, or chewing.

■ The person with a unilateral hearing loss should keep his or her good ear facing the speaker whenever possible.

■ If possible, avoid rooms with poor acoustics. If meetings are held in such rooms, request that they be transferred to better rooms. Special amplifications such as induction loops, radio-frequency hearing aids, or infrared devices are very useful in such situations.

■ Come early to meetings so you can sit close to the speaker.

■ When going to a movie or a play, read the reviews or a summary of the plot in advance.

■ In an extremely noisy situation, converse before the noise starts or after it ends.

Source: From Wayner, D., & Abrahamson, J. (1996). *Learning to Hear Again.* Austin, TX: Hear Again Publishing. Reprinted with permission.

APPENDIX 8–L

Communication Guidelines

For Listeners with Hearing Loss
1. Pick the best spot to communicate by avoiding areas that are poorly lit and very noisy.
2. Do not bluff!
3. Pay attention to the speaker.
4. Provide feedback that you understand or fail to understand.
5. Look for visual clues to what is being said.
6. Anticipate difficult situations and plan how to minimize problems.
7. Tell others how best to talk to you.
8. Provide feedback to speakers by saying how well they are doing.
9. Try not to interrupt too often.
10. Arrange for frequent breaks if discussions or meetings are long.
11. Set realistic goals about what you can expect to understand.
12. Ask for written clues of key words, if needed.

For Speakers
1. Get the person's attention before you speak.
2. Speak clearly and at a moderate pace.
3. Don't shout.
4. Avoid noisy background situations.
5. Rephrase when you are not understood.
6. Give clues when changing the subject.
7. Use facial expressions and gestures.
8. Be patient, positive, and relaxed.
9. Don't put objects in front of your face.
10. Do not have objects in your mouth such as gum, cigarettes, or food.
11. When in doubt, ask the hard of hearing person for suggestions to improve communications.
12. The person who begins a conversation must go to the listener.

(Based on Trychin, S., & Boone, M. (1987). *Communication Rules for Hard of Hearing People*, Bethesda, MD: SHHH Press)
Source: From Wayner, D., & Abrahamson, J. (1996). *Learning to Hear Again*. Austin, TX: Hear Again Publishing. Reprinted with permission.

APPENDIX 8–M

Rules for Good Communication

1. Indicate if you are not understanding.

2. Speak slightly louder, clearly, and slowly.

3. Speak to others as you want others to speak to you.

4. Determine the topic of conversation.

5. Position yourself for good communication.

6. Be creative and assertive in solving communication problems.

7. Look and listen for key words and phrases.

8. Plan ahead for difficult listening situations.

9. Take responsibility for communicating effectively.

Source: From Wayner, D., & Abrahamson, J. (1996). *Learning to Hear Again.* Austin, TX: Hear Again Publishing. Reprinted with permission.

APPENDIX 8–N

Basic Rules for Speechreading

■ Ask people to repeat if you do not understand them. Search for clues before you guess. Always indicate when you have not heard what has been said. Don't bluff!

■ Watch the speaker carefully so that you can see his/her total expression; it will give you a clue to what the speaker is saying. Don't concentrate on the speaker's lips alone; be aware of gestures, facial expressions, and body movements.

■ Check the seating arrangement in the room, and seat yourself in a seat across from the speaker so you can see his face. Be sure you are both in a good light. If you have difficulty seeing, move.

■ Determine, as soon as possible, what the topic of conversations is— even if you have to ask someone.

■ Look for ideas rather than for isolated words.

■ Relax while you are speechreading; try not to strain.

■ Keep abreast of current events so that you can enter into conversation.

■ Keep informed of your friends' interests and new developments so you will have something to talk about with them.

■ Tell your friends you are hearing impaired and are studying speechreading. Encourage them to help. (Ask them not to shout or exaggerate their words and ask that one person speak at a time.)

■ When asking for repetitions, repeat what you did get from the conversation so you can determine if you are on the right train of thought.

■ Don't worry that people think you are staring at them while you are speechreading. If this is a concern, tell them what you are doing.

■ Don't mouth words or sounds you see.

■ Pay attention to your speech. Since you might not always hear correctly, you might have a tendency to drop the ends of your words or to slur your words. Don't let your own speech become sloppy. Ask family and friends to help you monitor your speech.

- Remember that it takes time to become a good speechreader. Each individual will learn at his own rate. Plan to take repeated refresher courses during the years ahead.

- Don't be afraid of speechreading. It takes lots of practice, but once you begin using it, you will find that it is a good friend.

Source: From Wayner, D., & Abrahamson, J. (1996). *Learning to Hear Again.* Austin, TX: Hear Again Publishing. Reprinted with permission.

APPENDIX 8–O

10 Keys to Effective Listening

Keys to Effective Listening	The Bad Listener	The Good Listener
1. Find areas of interest	Tunes out dry subjects	Opportunizes & asks "What's in it for me?"
2. Judge content, not delivery	Tunes out if delivery is poor	Judges content, skips over delivery errors
3. Hold your fire!	Tends to enter into argument	Doesn't judge until comprehension complete
4. Listen for ideas	Listens for facts	Listens for central themes
5. Be flexible	Takes intensive notes	Takes fewer notes
6. Work at listening	Shows no energy output	Works hard, exhibits active body state
7. Resist distractions	Distracted easily	Fights or avoids distractions, tolerates bad habits, knows how to concentrate
8. Exercise your mind	Resists difficult material; seeks light material	Uses heavier material as exercise for the mind
9. Keep your mind open	Reacts to emotional words	Interprets color words; does not get hung up on them
10. Capitalize on fact thought is faster than speech	Tends to daydream with slow speakers	Challenges, anticipates, summarizes, weighs the evidence, listens between the lines to tone of voice

Source: From Wayner, D., & Abrahamson, J. (1996). *Learning to Hear Again.* Austin, TX: Hear Again Publishing. Reprinted with permission.

APPENDIX 8–P

Good Communication Involves ACTION

There are many things that individuals with hearing loss can do in order to take the best advantage of state-of-the-art hearing instruments. Actions by their frequent communication partners can also go a long way in reducing the communication and interpersonal challenges that can go along with hearing loss.

The Listener can:

- **Pay attention:** Concentration is very important

- **Develop good listening skills:** Concentrate on what is said.

- **Observe the talker:** What you see can supplement what you hear.

- **Plan ahead:** Think about possible challenges to clear understanding you may face. Plan what to do if they occur.

- **Take breaks if needed:** Listening with a hearing loss can be tiring. You can concentrate better if you are fresh.

- **Make specific suggestions about how to talk to you:** For example, it is better to ask a person to rephrase or slow down rather than just say "What?"

- **Provide feedback:** If you tell your partner what you heard, both of you will know right away if you understood correctly.

- **Double check details:** Repeating what you understood someone to say can prevent confusion later on, especially dates and times.

- **Do not bluff!** Pretending you understand when you don't is a "no-win" situation.

- **Set realistic expectations:** Some situations are just too noisy to expect to understand clearly even with the best hearing aids.

Source: From Wayner, D., & Abrahamson, J. (1996). *Learning to Hear Again.* Austin, TX: Hear Again Publishing. Reprinted with permission.

APPENDIX 8–Q

Twelve Listening Tips

1. Relearn the trick of concentration. Pay attention. Listen.

2. Avoid pretending that you have understood what was said. It will only confuse things later.

3. Don't be afraid to ask people to repeat or speak up louder.

4. Don't hesitate to inform the speaker that you have a hearing impairment and suggest what he or she can do to help you hear better.

5. Remind people to speak to you.

6. Carefully watch the speaker. Attend to the lips, facial expressions and gestures, and body language.

7. Position yourself to take advantage of good lighting. Have the light come from behind you. Rearrange your position if you find that there is a glare on the speaker's face. This will assist you in using all nonverbal cues.

8. At informal gatherings, try to limit the number of people you speak with at one time. One-to-one conversations are easier than group conversations.

9. Hearing in noisy places is a problem for all listeners. At parties, meetings, theater, movies, and church, practice will help you learn to separate speech from background noise.

10. Encourage the use of public address systems at meetings or at church, when they are available.

11. Try to arrive early at large group functions so that you can have the option of sitting close to the speaker(s). Position yourself in the best situation to hear as well as see.

12. When listening over the telephone, use the T-switch (if applicable) and place the receiver close to the microphone.

Source: From Wayner, D., & Abrahamson, J. (1996). *Learning to Hear Again.* Austin, TX: Hear Again Publishing. Reprinted with permission.

APPENDIX 8–R

Suggestions for Improving Communication by Being Assertive for People With Hearing Loss

Three ways to react to difficult communication situations are to be:

Passive:

- Withdraws from communication situations thus avoiding misunderstanding or conflicts
- Reacts by smiling, nodding the head, and pretending to understand
- Results in poor communication

Aggressive:

- Expresses feelings and needs openly in such a way that violates the other person's rights
- Reacts in a hostile manner to the speaker
- Refuses to admit even partial responsibility for communication breakdowns—all blame placed on other person
- Dominates conversations
- Results in no real communication exchange

Assertive:

- Admits their problems and asks for assistance
- Takes initiative for improving the communication situation
- Respects their partner's and their own needs for communication to happen
- Results in good communication exchange

Source: From Wayner, D., & Abrahamson, J. (1996). *Learning to Hear Again*. Austin, TX: Hear Again Publishing. Reprinted with permission.

APPENDIX 8–S

Assistive Devices for Persons with Hearing Impairment

Alerting Devices

Visual

Call Alert
Ring Indicator / Lamp
Rotating Beacon
Strobe Light
Flasher Button
Phone Flash / Strobe
Clock Radio with Outlet Plug
Baby Cry
Knock Light

Auditory

Ring Max
Fone Alert
Loud Ringer
Buzzer
Gong
Rodelvox

Tactile

Shake / Awake
Pillow Vibrator
Bed Vibrator
Fan
Quest, Tactaid
Hearing Dogs
Wrist Vibrator
Quiet Wake

Telephone Amplification and Aids

Portable Amplifier
Handset Amplifier
Telelink
Whistle Stop
Telephone Typewriter
Relay System
Earpads for Receiver

Television Amplification and Aids

Sound Jacks
Amplified Speaker
Transistor Radio / TV Band
Closed Caption Decoder
Personal Listening Extension Cord
Pocketalker
Stereo Amplified Listener
Infrared Transmitter / Receiver

Personal One-to-One Communication

Pockettalker
FM System
Amplified Listener

Large Area Listening

Infra-Red System
Induction Loops
Noise Buster
FM System / Personal Receivers
Transistor Radio / Headset or Ear Buds

Source: From Wayner, D., & Abrahamson, J. (1996). *Learning to Hear Again.* Austin, TX: Hear Again Publishing. Reprinted with permission.

APPENDIX 8–T

Types of Coping

Emotion-Focused Coping (feeling better) (based on Trychin, S., 1987)
- Escape Avoidance Behaviors
- Frustration-withdrawal-depression
- Thoughts and realistic expectations

Problem-Focused Coping Strategies (solving the problem) (based on Kaplan, H. et al, 1985)
- Anticipatory strategies
  - Anticipate possible vocabulary
  - Anticipate possible dialogue and its sequences
  - Anticipate questions that may be asked and decide what information is needed
  - Plan questions to ask
  - Decide how to narrow and specify questions
  - Anticipate environmental problems
  - Plan how to modify the environment
  - Consider how to be assertive without being overbearing
- Repair strategies
  - Rephrase
  - Say key words
  - Summarize
  - Spell key word
  - Say each number individually
  - Ask a specific question
  - Ask a general question
  - Write a brief message (focus on key words)
  - Gesture
  - Let people know what you need
    - Tell them clearly and simply what they need to do
    - Provide opportunities for them to practice correct behavior
    - Provide feedback about how well they are doing

Source: From Wayner, D., & Abrahamson, J. (1996). *Learning to Hear Again.* Austin, TX: Hear Again Publishing. Reprinted with permission.

Up to this point in the book, we have dealt primarily with patients who, given proper counseling, are at least capable of understanding the importance of trying, and hopefully succeeding, with the integration of hearing aids into the process of improved communication. In the final two chapters, our attention is directed toward other challenging segments of the hearing impaired population. In Chapter 9, Becky Bingea describes many of the approaches and modifications to traditional counseling and orientation that are required when dealing with parents of children who are hearing impaired. For these cases, not only must the emotions, resistance, and education of the patient be attended to, but also many of these issues must be approached indirectly through third parties, many of whom bring along their own set of problems. Because serving the pediatric population frequently requires multidisciplinary assistance, and because of the demand for additional pediatric services, an extensive list of reading materials, resources, support services, and laws governing education of hearing impaired children is provided in the Appendixes.

9

Challenges in Counseling Parents of Children With Hearing Loss

■ Becky Bingea, M.A. ■

Inherent in successful amplification of children with hearing loss is the support, understanding, and follow-through of the parents. Just as counseling adult patients is a professional responsibility of the audiologist, so, too, is counseling the parents and families of children who have hearing loss. This can be quite challenging, but it can also be very rewarding. The counseling process may be most intense during and immediately following the identification of hearing loss, but should be considered an ongoing process that will involve the child, the child's parents and family, and other professionals who work with the child. Different challenges will arise at different stages. At each stage, the process will be enhanced by respect, trust, and adherence to the basic tenets of good communication and by working as a team with the parents, child, family, and other involved professionals.

THE INITIAL INTERACTION AND DIAGNOSIS

Accurate diagnosis of hearing loss and preparation of the parents and family is necessary in order to move toward successful intervention

263

with amplification. Initial counseling interactions go a long way toward parent acceptance of the diagnosis and the child's future success with hearing aids.

Conducting the Initial Diagnostic Interaction

First impressions are important in gaining the trust and commitment of the child's parents and family and, as noted by Johnson (1997), "usually set the tone for subsequent interactions" (p. 18). These first impressions will be influenced by the physical environment, the ability of the audiologist to demonstrate professional competence and confidence, and sincere interest in and respect for the family.

First impressions are enhanced by a positive physical environment, including waiting room, testing, and counseling areas that are arranged for comfort and ease of communication. For example:

- Is there ample seating?
- Is the office staff open and friendly?
- Are the rooms disorganized or sterile-looking, or are they tidy and comfortable?
- Is the environment "child-friendly"?
- Are the parents easily able to participate in or observe the testing?
- Is seating arranged for counseling such that eye contact and verbal and nonverbal interaction is enhanced?
- Is there an alternate supervised room or adjacent area in which the young child can be entertained or distracted while discussing sensitive issues with the parents?

Professional competence is demonstrated through verbal and nonverbal presentation and interaction, including directness of questions and answers, vocal tone and rate, eye contact, and body language. Preparation for the appointment by reviewing all available information about the child and having needed test instruments and materials at hand allows a smooth transition and flow into the history-taking, testing, and counseling. Eye contact and interaction should be maintained with both parents and any other family members present. How the audiologist is dressed and seated (poised yet comfortable? attentive and interested?) may also affect the parents' perception of professionalism.

Focusing first on the parents' questions and concerns in the intake interview and history-taking, and listening with care and concern in a nonjudgmental manner, show respect for their viewpoints, ideas, observations, and prior experiences. It also gives the parents a sense of control and allows the audiologist to gain their confidence and important information that may not otherwise have been offered. Listen to or look for what is *not* being said (through body language or covert meanings) as well as to what *is* said. For example, one parent may say, "My wife thinks he's not responding, but I think he's okay," but another set of parents might just exchange looks when asked if there are any concerns about their child's hearing.

It can be helpful to prepare the parents prior to onset of the testing that more than one session may be needed before a diagnosis can be provided. Because young or delayed children do not always perform optimally in a new environment, in a testing situation, or at a given time, pieces of information to obtain the complete (or at least preliminary) diagnosis may need to be collected across sessions. As discussed later, even when a preliminary definition of hearing loss is obtained, the diagnostic process with the hearing-impaired child is ongoing as hearing status becomes further defined.

Including the parents in the actual diagnostic process by having them present in the test room (e.g., sitting with or behind their child) or observing during the testing demonstrates respect for the importance of their involvement. It also demonstrates to them how their child does or does not respond, which can lead to a better understanding and acceptance of the diagnosis to follow.

Presenting the Diagnosis, Implications, and Recommendations

In presenting the diagnosis, implications, and recommendations, the sophistication of the parents, their ability to understand and follow through, their stage in the grieving process, and their cultural backgrounds must be considered.

How to Present the Information

The amount, type, and detail of information presented to the parents at the initial appointment will vary from family to family and according to the degree of hearing loss. It is important to monitor the parents' reactions and understanding throughout this interaction to determine how much information and detail is sufficient. The parents may be overwhelmed by the information being provided and its emotional impact, even if the diagnosis was anticipated, rendering them unable to attend to or comprehend much of what is said after the diagnosis. Addressing the parents' questions and concerns right away with direct and honest answers may allow them to "hear" other things that are presented to them. The parents should be assured that they may call, as well as return, to further discuss the information presented and any additional questions they might have.

As in the initial interview, the audiologist may need to respond to covert meanings (what is actually said may not be what is actually meant or asked), and both verbal and nonverbal messages must be examined. A parent who quickly responds, "Yea, yea, I know what you mean," while packing up jackets and belongings, may not really have understood, may not want to admit he didn't understand, may be indicating unwillingness to learn anything further, or may not be able to cope with the situation at the moment. The approach used with a parent who reacts to information with a smirk or inattention will likely be different than that used with a parent who has tears welling up.

In responding to parent reactions and emotions, it is important to *empathize with* rather than *sympathize for* the parents. Rather than patronizing the parents or "feeling sorry" for them, listen in a warm and caring manner, validate their feelings, have an understanding of the grieving process, and communicate the results with respect and sensitivity. Empathy involves an understanding of what the parents are going through (without necessarily having to go through it yourself) and communicating that awareness. Attentive behavior, eye contact, warm or concerned facial expressions, vocal tone, body posture, and physical proximity communicate the audiologist's interest and involvement. (A box of tissues nearby is often helpful, too!) Diefendorf et al. (1990) noted that it may be easier for the audiologist to focus on the technical information, but at this point, counseling and emotional support is vital. They advised the audiologist to "keep in mind that at that moment they [the parents] are the most important people in the world—and their child is the most important child in the world" (p. 394).

Because of the necessary emphasis on the diagnosis, there is also a tendency to focus on "impairment," forgetting to provide encouragement by accentuating the child's and parents' assets. Maintaining a positive, optimistic counseling environment includes sharing with the parents observations and reports of their child's strengths. For example, the explanation of the results may begin by relating how well the child behaved and interacted in the test environment, how reliably the child responded, or how quickly the child learned the test task (provided these were truly observed, of course). The parents' sense of control, self-esteem, and self-confidence should be enhanced by seeking and stressing the importance of their advice and observations, and also by sharing observations of positive directions and appropriate steps they are already taking (e.g., their communicative interactions with their child or their endeavors to seek and find appropriate intervention for their child). It should be emphasized, however, that a positive approach does not mean discounting or minimizing the grief and sadness the parents may be experiencing, no matter what degree of hearing loss is present.

It is important to be aware that the parents may not be ready to accept the diagnosis at this point. An understanding of the grieving process, including common reactions of pain, denial, anger, fear, guilt, confusion, avoidance, and rationalization helps the professional deal with this phase. This involves accepting the parents' feelings as normal human reactions without taking their emotional responses personally. Express your understanding and support in a way that might encourage parents to voice their concerns and emotions, and let them know that they are not alone (e.g., "How are you feeling about all of this?" or, "I have found that parents often feel overwhelmed by this information").

Although fear of the unknown is often more difficult for parents than fearing what is known (i.e., having the diagnosis of hearing loss, which may give them direction), parents will likely fear the future: "Will he eventually lose all of his hearing?" "Will he have to learn sign language?" "Should *we* learn sign language?" "Will he learn to talk?" These questions must be addressed and explained clearly when providing information about the hearing loss and its implications. The emotional burden can be eased by encouraging the parents to discuss the diagnosis with each other, their families, religious advisors, close friends, and other persons significant in their lives. Putting the parents in touch with other parents of children who are hearing impaired can be especially helpful at this point.

A parent not yet ready to accept the diagnosis might ask, "Couldn't he just be congested today? He has a cold." The audiologist could then respond: "That's a very good question. That's why we performed a special test to assess that part of the ear. It showed us that there is no congestion in his ear right now." Parents may not be ready to accept the diagnosis because they are confused by the results: "How come her speech is fine?" or, "How could she possibly hear the garbage truck coming down the street before any of the rest of us?" or, "Wouldn't we have noticed if she had a hearing loss?" Careful presentation of the results to explain what appears to be inconsistency between the results and what the parents have observed is very important, and is discussed in a later section. Confusion may also be apparent when a parent doesn't truly process or fully accept what is being said: "So, his hearing isn't really that bad, is it?" or, "But he doesn't really need hearing aids, right?"

Parents who react to the diagnosis with anger directed toward the professional are likely trying to cope with the loss of their "perfect" child and, perhaps, with guilt from the possibility that they may have caused their child's hearing loss ("I shouldn't have taken that drug during my pregnancy") or that they delayed the diagnosis ("I should have known he was not hearing"). The parents, at this point, may request a second opinion. This is not necessarily a reflection on the services that have been provided but, rather, their need to confirm the diagnosis or, perhaps, their quest to regain their "normal" child. Luterman (1985) pointed out that denial is a way of coping with grief and, until the parents have other ways of coping, they may not be able to give up their denial. Accepting or even encouraging the parents' desire to obtain another opinion, rather than becoming defensive about it, acknowledges their feelings at the moment, helps them feel some sense of control of the process, and may allow them to move forward sooner than they otherwise would. It may also increase their confidence in the audiologist who trusts her own results enough to encourage assessment elsewhere.

In responding to perceptions of parent denial, Luterman (1985) cautioned professionals to leave alone "positive denial" that can give parents a source of strength (e.g., the optimism from hoping for an eventual cure) and to not be too quick to label parent responses as "denial" when, in fact, they may be legitimate differences of opinion.

As cultural diversity in this country increases, there is a need to be aware of differences in attitudes toward hearing loss and intervention. For example, some cultures may view hearing loss as a sign of infirmity or weakness; the parents may not want to discuss their child's hearing loss further or call attention to it in any way, particularly with hearing aids. An understanding of hierarchical positions in family roles and responsibilities enables the audiologist to modify the approach with certain families *before* trying a usual approach and not succeeding. A knowledgeable foreign-language interpreter outside of the family can often provide invaluable assistance in understanding another culture, in anticipating potential responses from the family, in "reading" the parents' responses to the situation, and in planning a course of action with a specific family.

To Whom to Present the Information

Both Parents. Because one parent may be more willing to accept the diagnosis and recommendations than the other, it is very important to include both parents (again, verbally and nonverbally) as much as possible in the testing, diagnosis, counseling, and eventual intervention process. It also helps to have more than one person listen to the same information, as one parent or family member may have stopped listening after the diagnosis was made or the words "hearing aids" were mentioned. Furthermore, one parent may not remember something that the other parent did.

Traditionally mothers have provided much of the emotional support and have attended to their children when they are ill, need appointments, and so forth. Although these trends are changing as lifestyle attitudes have changed and more mothers have entered the work force, our culture has been one in which fathers may react and interact differently with their children and the professionals working with them than do mothers (Rushmer, 1994). However, this is no reason to exclude fathers from the process. In fact, a father's participation in and support for the entire process are strongly encouraged.

Anger and denial may be stronger in the parent not present to participate in the diagnostic and habilitative process. Parental involvement and support necessitates inclusion of both parents as much as possible. If only one parent is present at the time of diagnosis, invite that parent to return with the other parent to discuss the findings and implications again.

The Child Who is Hearing Impaired. Depending on the child's age, the child may or may not be included in the initial discussion of the results, implications, and recommendations. Unless the child is older, it is probably not appropriate to include the child in all aspects of the counseling sessions. It is important to have the parents' full attention during counseling, without distractions from the child. Also, the child may feel guilty about his parent crying or expressing distress or anger, feeling that he has caused the parent to react that way. The parents need to be able to project a positive, upbeat attitude to let the child know that he did not do anything wrong and that the hearing loss does not make him "bad."

However, a child who is not included at all in discussions may also feel he is "bad" or has done something wrong. The child must be included in some way at some time in order to gain trust in and the desire to work with the audiologist to achieve the agreed upon goals. Use of pictures or examples to illustrate something just related to the parents will enhance the child's understanding. If the younger child is not present during emotional discussions with the parents, the audiologist can later attend to the child with pictures, sample hearing aids, and/or simple explanations of how she will be working with him to hear new sounds. If it is not possible to discuss all issues with the parents because of the child's presence, a follow-up session without the child or a phone call should be arranged.

Including the older child who is hearing impaired, especially an adolescent or teenager, in decisions about intervention and amplification will enhance understanding and cooperation. Although it is less likely that a hearing loss will be identified at this age, the possibility of progressive or late-onset hearing loss does, of course, exist. Even a child identified earlier will likely want and need to become more involved as he gets older. It is important to remember that children, not only parents, need to grieve, too. Children of all ages need to be supported by their parents and others around them in their efforts to cope with their hearing loss and the changes it will create in their lives. Parents may try to comfort their child by pointing out how another child they know overcame an illness; but the teenager may point out that his loss is different because it's permanent and he has to live with it forever. This should be acknowledged as true, but that it's only a part of who he is; it doesn't have to exist out of proportion to other parts of him. This is not always easy to grasp or accept at first (possibly never for some), but providing tools for support will help. For example, the audiologist or parent may say:

> "It's true that you will have to live with it, and it *is* a part of you. But it's not the only part of you. People will notice if you have a new shirt and you may say, 'Thanks, I just got it last weekend,' or may comment on your haircut, and you may say, 'Yea, I'm trying a new style.' They will also notice your hearing aids and you can acknowledge that, too, and say, 'Yea, and now I can hear better.' Once you explain it to them, they will be more likely to move on."

Siblings and Other Family Members.   It is important to include siblings and other family members or care workers involved with the child. If they are not present at the initial session, attempts should be made to include them later in some way, whether directly or through the parents. Family relationships may suffer if attention is focused on the child with hearing loss, to the exclusion of siblings. Conversely, siblings who *are* included and viewed as important, and who are also given their own special attention, can enhance family interactions and follow-through. The more the family and extended family understands, the more likely they are to be helpful and support the intervention process.

What Information to Present

As previously discussed, the amount of information that can be presented at the initial session will be limited by the ability of the parents to accept the diagnosis and their ability to understand what, to them, will likely be a bombardment of technical information at a time when they may be emotionally fragile. A series of appointments is recommended in order to convey the information and counsel the parents appropriately. Early on, however, the parents should be educated in an unbiased manner in the areas to follow so that they have a good understanding of their child's hearing loss and its implications to allow them to make appropriate choices for intervention. They also need to know that their choices in the beginning may not be their choices later on; they have the right to change their minds as they gather new information and evaluate how their child is progressing. For some parents, counseling during the initial session may involve only the diagnosis and an outline or mention of some of the other items. For other parents, the explanations and discussion may be more detailed. Regardless of how quickly this happens, ongoing monitoring of parent comprehension is vital, as is arranging follow-up sessions during which further information can be provided and assimilated at a pace the parents can handle successfully.

Type and Degree of Hearing Loss and Possible Cause(s).

- Explain the hearing loss and its implications in language that the parents can understand.
- Provide concrete evidence of the hearing loss rather than abstract references, and demonstrate if necessary. If a parent is present in the test booth during the testing, he or she will likely experience what the child could and could not hear. Later when hearing aids are fitted, parents may relate to the child's hearing loss further by observing aided and unaided responses in the sound booth. In addition, when explaining the audiogram, parents can listen through earphones to various frequencies and hearing levels. Use of videos, pictures, diagrams, and tapes or CDs with filtered speech or simulated hearing loss can also be helpful in illustrating the verbal presentation.
- Compare the hearing loss with normal hearing.
- Explain whether the hearing loss is permanent, temporary, or fluctuating. Parents often wonder if their child who is hearing impaired but not deaf will become deaf. Parents also may assume the hearing loss is temporary and that the child will "grow out of it." Even children often assume, on their own, that they will no longer have hearing loss when they grow up.
- Explain the educational implications of the hearing loss and implications for speech and language. Parents of children with severe-to-profound hearing loss often wonder if their child will learn to speak.

It is important to emphasize that many variables are involved, including the amount of residual hearing, amplification, educational program, parental involvement, timeliness of intervention, and the child (cognitive potential, other disabilities, etc.).

Amplification Options.

- Explain and show the types of hearing aids and what's appropriate for the particular child and hearing loss.
- Stress and explain the importance of binaural amplification, unless there is clearly no usable hearing in one ear or there are obvious tolerance problems.
- Discuss the potential benefits and limitations of hearing aids and of assistive listening devices, such as FM systems.
- Discuss the possibility of a cochlear implant if the hearing loss is severe to profound, especially if the parents desire a strong aural/oral program component for their child.

Educational Options.

- Provide information and resources regarding oral/auditory, Auditory-Verbal, American Sign Language (ASL), cued speech, total communication, and combination options, such as a bilingual-bicultural-bimodal approach, in an impartial way.
- Provide information on residential versus nonresidential options.
- Be aware of personal biases toward intervention. If those biases do not allow all options to be presented in a thorough manner, refer the parents to someone who can convey the options.

Importance of Timely Intervention.

- Explain the benefits of early intervention and timely follow-up. Be aware that the parents may not be able to move as quickly as desirable. Because their cooperation is needed and intervention won't get far without them, the process may need to move at a slower pace that the parents can handle.
- Provide resources and tools for education and involvement even if the parents may not yet be ready to follow through.
- Even with the benefits of early intervention, discuss (or reinforce from the earlier discussion on hearing loss implications) realistic expectations regarding auditory responsiveness and speech and language.

Hearing Health Care.

■ Refer the child for medical/otologic evaluation to rule out structural lesions and syndromic or other medical problems, including visual, cardiac, metabolic, kidney, and immunologic disorders.

■ Recommend genetic evaluation and counseling. Although the otologist or pediatrician will often make this referral, be aware that the audiologist's responsibility is not relinquished if another professional does not make the referral. Professionals may be held liable for not informing parents that there can be a genetic component to hearing loss. On the other hand, it is important to be cautious in how this recommendation is presented to avoid making judgments about parents' decisions to have future children who may be hearing impaired. Genetic evaluation is used to try to determine the cause of the hearing loss and whether it is genetic or environmental. If it is determined to be genetic, the pattern of inheritance and the probability of future children inheriting hearing loss is explained. Genetic counselors do not advise families whether to have future children, but rather provide education regarding the cause of the hearing loss and information regarding medical and support services (Arnos, Downs, Israel, & Cunningham, 1989).

■ Provide information on the dangers of exposure to loud noise and the use of ear protection.

■ Provide information about ear infections and the importance of prompt medical attention to prevent structural damage as well as compromised residual hearing from a conductive overlay.

■ Provide information on safety issues related to the possibility of not hearing danger signals in the environment, and the importance of using vision to supplement any auditory cues.

Emotional/Psychosocial Health Care.

■ Be familiar with psychiatric diagnostic categories and signs of social/psychological/emotional problems (of the child and parents) beyond the audiologist's scope of practice and expertise.

■ Be alert to parents or families (including the child) who are not progressing through the grieving process or who are exhibiting unhealthy or unproductive family dynamics in dealing with the child's hearing loss.

■ When indicated, provide the parents with referrals for emotional/psychosocial services.

Closing the Initial Session

At the end of the session, the parents should be given written or pictorial information, including literature on hearing loss, hearing aids, and educational options. Tapes and videos may also be helpful. Awareness of local resources is vital in practicing pediatric audiology. Provide a list of resources, such as medical referrals, parent groups, educational services, speech-language pathologists, and financial resources. Not only do these materials reinforce the information provided during the session, but they give the parents tools for taking an active role in their child's intervention. The Appendixes at the end of this chapter provide specific resource suggestions. As stated previously, the specific amount of the information that may be given to the parents in the first session will vary from family to family according to their immediate concerns and how much they can reasonably handle. The ability to judge this evolves as the audiologist gains experience in counseling.

Maintaining confidentiality of patient records is a professional and legal responsibility. Signed "Release and Exchange of Information" forms should be explained and obtained in order to make referrals to or receive information from other agencies or individuals.

Before leaving, the parents should be given an idea of what happens next and a preliminary time line for follow-up. They should also be given information on how to reach the audiologist and be encouraged to call should questions or concerns arise prior to the next appointment.

The child and parents deserve every opportunity for success. Each audiologist must be aware of her limitations. If a high quality service cannot be provided, the family should be referred to another audiologist.

FOLLOW-UP AFTER THE INITIAL DIAGNOSIS AND COUNSELING

A first follow-up appointment should be scheduled soon after the initial diagnosis for further testing to confirm and/or expand upon the test results. Additionally, this appointment is important to provide an opportunity for continued counseling and ongoing education and support to the parents by reviewing information given to them previously, checking for their understanding and comprehension (e.g., asking them to explain their understanding of the hearing loss), checking for any obstacles to their progress, and answering any questions. Information may need to be reviewed over several follow-up sessions. Additional written information may be provided, if needed. The time interval for this first follow-up appointment will necessarily vary depending on the parents' and audiologist's schedules, financial authorization arrangements, geographic accessibility, and so forth, but preferably within 1 to 2 weeks.

Discussion at the follow-up appointments includes reiteration or further explanation of the importance of ongoing audiological/hearing aid monitoring and the ongoing nature of diagnosis and intervention. There is typically refinement of test results over time as the child becomes accustomed to the testing tasks and to using auditory information. Responses to test stimuli often improve after the child has gained increased experience with auditory input (Diefendorf et al., 1990; Stelmachowicz, Larson, Johnson, & Moeller, 1985). It is important to check the stability of the hearing loss over time to monitor for progressive hearing loss and also the possibility of fluctuations from ear infections to which younger children may be especially prone. Once the child has hearing aids, follow-up is important for monitoring earmold fit in the growing child, hearing aid function and benefit, loudness discomfort, and educational and developmental progress. Parent observations and input are vital in providing appropriate follow-up.

The frequency of follow-up appointments will depend on the reliability of the test results, the child's developmental level and attention span (how much can be accomplished in a given session), the stability of the hearing loss, and how recent the diagnosis. Although follow-up will vary according to these individual factors, a general recommendation, as suggested by Stelmachowicz et al. (1985), would be every 3 to 4 months for children up to 3 years old, every 6 months for children 3 to 6 years old, and at least annually for school-age children over 6 years old.

HEARING AID ORIENTATION: COUNSELING ON HEARING AID USE AND CARE

As with adults, hearing aid orientation and counseling is essential to successful hearing aid use for children. The difference, of course, is that children often do not or cannot offer feedback to the audiologist; therefore, the audiologist must rely on the accuracy of the information provided by the parents. It is important that parents have a good understanding of amplification and its related issues to ensure that hearing aids are providing appropriate and consistent benefit. Parents may become overwhelmed at this stage, as well, but by providing simple, clear instructions that are reinforced with written and pictorial handouts, many parents become relative experts in a short period of time.

General Orientation

A brief orientation to the parts of hearing aids and their functions helps to put the remainder of the discussion in perspective. Diagrams from user booklets will remind the parents of these parts if they do not remember them. Troubleshooting of the hearing aids and counseling regarding cleaning and care of the aids and earmolds should be reviewed verbally and supplemented with take-home written information. Provision of a parent hearing aid care kit is vital to facilitate maintenance and monitoring of hearing aid function. (See the listing of suggested items in Appendix 9–A.) Battery caution should be stressed along with provision of the number for the National Button Battery Ingestion Hotline. Tamper-resistant battery doors and volume-control covers are useful for small children and should be explained to the parents. Hearing aid warranties should be carefully reviewed, along with options for extended warranties for repair and loss/damage. These options can be discussed in greater detail at the end of the hearing aid trial period. Although many adults may opt not to purchase extended warranties for their own hearing aids, it is prudent to recommend extended warranties for children's hearing aids because children can be very hard on hearing aids and loss is common.

Initially, parents may be afraid to handle the hearing aids. Hearing aids should be handled with care, but they must be handled to be used! Encouraging the parents to manipulate the hearing aids during orientation assists in overcoming this initial fear of "doing something wrong" or breaking the hearing aids.

Daily Hearing Aid Checks and Care

Daily visual and listening checks are important and should be stressed. Studies consistently demonstrate high rates of hearing aid malfunction when sampled in schools (Elfenbein, Bentler, Davis, & Niebuhr, 1988). A demonstration of how to listen to the hearing aids through a stethoscope from the parent kit can be provided, with an explanation to the parents that, although the hearing aids may sound strange to them at first, as they listen daily, they will become accustomed to how they *should* sound and will then be likely to hear the difference if a malfunction occurs. Listening through the earmold will allow the parents to make sure the entire system (earmold and hearing aid) is functioning, because they may not readily see moisture or cracking in the tubing that could impair hearing aid benefit. Daily checks can become quick and automatic if the parents have a routine to learn and follow. Simple instructions can be given to the parents to help them get started.

An example of these steps for a *preschooler* (with modifications individualized to each child's specific hearing aid controls and prescribed settings) might be as follows:

DAILY HEARING AID STEPS

Morning
1. Check hearing aid batteries with the battery tester. If the batteries are not working, replace them with fresh ones. Do not let your child watch you change the batteries.
2. Insert the batteries, making sure the polarity is correct (positive matches positive) and shut the battery door.
3. Visually inspect the casing and earhooks of the hearing aids for any cracking or damage.
4. For each hearing aid, attach the listening tube or stethoscope to the earmold of the hearing aid. Listen to the hearing aid through the earmold as you speak and rotate the volume control. Listen for any scratchiness, breaks in the signal, or distortion. If the sound is not normal, detach the earmold and attach the stethoscope to the earhook of the hearing aid and listen to the hearing aid again. If the sound is now normal, the problem is likely with the earmold or earmold tubing. Check the earmold to make sure there is no moisture or wax in the tubing or ports, cracks in the earmold or tubing, or crimping of the tubing.
5. Put the hearing aids on your child. Check the earmold fit. Turn the hearing aids on ("M" position), and adjust the volume controls to #2.
6. Listen for any feedback ("whistling") when the hearing aids are properly in place. This may indicate the need for new earmolds.

Break time
1. Turn the hearing aids off ("O" position), remove, and place them in their cases in a safe location out of the reach of children or animals and away from excessive heat or moisture.
2. Check your child's ears for any signs of redness or irritation.

Bedtime
1. Shut the hearing aids off ("O" position) and take them out.
2. Check the earmolds and clean with a tissue or damp cloth and tools (i.e., brush and wax loop) if necessary, to remove wax. If

Continued

they are particularly waxy or dirty, disconnect the earmolds from the hearing aids to wash them, but do not get the hearing aid wet. Use the forced-air bulb to blow out any excess moisture from the earmolds and tubing. Check the earmold tubing for cracks, crimping, or brittleness.

3. Open the battery doors and place the hearing aids in their open boxes. (Let them "air out" over night.) Place the boxes in a safe location away from children and pets and away from excessive heat or moisture.

To avoid overwhelming parents at this first orientation, you may choose to give them only parts of the hearing aid care kit. For example, the dri-aid kit may not be critical the first week or two and can be reviewed at the next appointment.

Adjusting to Hearing Aid Use and Scheduling Wearing Time

Intuition and experience will eventually guide the audiologist's recommendations to the parents regarding initial use and adjustment to wearing hearing aids. Recommendations will be modified by both child and parent reactions. Clues for initial attitudes toward and acceptance of the hearing aids can often be observed in the office during the fitting and orientation. Consideration should be given to what the child and parents can handle without compromising use of the hearing aids.

General recommendations include a wearing schedule that will eventually, but gradually, work up to full-time use, preferably by the end of the first week or two, if not sooner. Avoid noisy environments at first. The initial exposure to loud sound can be frightening or disturbing to some children. Quiet, pleasant environments at home, and language-rich activities (e.g., reading books, playing quietly and talking about your activities, watching television, or listening to gentle music) are a good place to start. Make the experience a pleasant one. Some children, especially babies and toddlers, may need a very gradual increase in use initially (e.g., 10- to 30-minute periods on, 30 minutes off, adding 15 minutes/day to the wearing time of each session). Older children and some younger children may be content for longer periods of use, and many will be able to adapt to full-time use almost immediately. Although the goal is full-time use from the time the child gets up in the morning until bedtime, the process is not a race and should be a gentle and positive experience. It may be beneficial to advise parents to turn off and remove the hearing aids before the child becomes agitated, tired, or asks to have them removed. This recommendation must be considered on an individual basis, however, as it might encourage some parents to remove the hearing aids before the child wants or needs to remove them and may also provide the parents with an excuse to minimize wearing time because of their own difficulties accepting amplification. Wearing schedules may also need to be adjusted when family routines are significantly altered, for example, when the child is ill or when there is a house full of out-of-town guests.

The importance of eventual full-time use cannot to be overemphasized. The use of consistent amplification for maximum adjustment, benefit, and success with hearing aids should be stressed. Some parents may be under the impression that amplification is only important when the child is at school. However, much of our learning occurs incidentally and in "casual" environments of home and play, including recess, sports, and physical education, thus the hearing aids should be worn in these situations as well (provided that safety has been ensured). Soft earmolds with BTE hearing aids that are insured for repair and loss and damage are recommended so children *can* use their hearing aids full time during their waking hours. Super Seals (Just Bekuz Products) can help with moisture problems during physical exertion and can be ordered to match the child's school uniform. Because learning occurs in all environments, it is important to wear the hearing aids in all environments, unless there are compelling reasons not to.

Activities for Parent Observation and Parent/Child Interaction

In addition to parent involvement in taking care of the hearing aids and scheduling and monitoring their use, other parent activities, especially in the early stages of hearing aid use, can enhance the child's aural habilitation, fulfill the parents' desire to take an active role in their child's experience with and adjustment to hearing aids and audition, and provide the audiologist with information from which to make hearing aid adjustments (Stelmachowicz et al., 1985).

Information obtained from a parent journal or check-off boxes in a log as to when, where, and how long the child uses the hearing aids can be helpful. Written data regarding observations of the child's responsiveness allow the audiologist and the parents to track responsiveness and progress, as well as to detect potential problems. An example of a combination checklist and written log form is provided in Appendix 9–D of this chapter. Activities to elicit observations might include reciprocal vocal play (e.g., parents and child taking turns imitating sounds) or walking around the house and listening to household sounds with their child. The experience should be a positive and realistic one: never ask the child to listen for sounds that you're not sure he can hear. A "lotto" listening game, in which the child matches pictures to sounds that are heard, can be fun when the child is old enough.

Along with other activities, the use of more formal observation measures of hearing aid benefit can be completed by the parent (and child, depending on age) to assist the audiologist in counseling parents and obtaining information regarding hearing aid benefit. An example is the combined use of the Parent's Abbreviated Profile of Hearing Aid Performance (PA-PHAP) and the Children's Abbreviated Profile of Hearing Aid Performance (CA-PHAP) that were adapted by audiologists at Boys Town National Research Hospital (Kopun & Stelmachowicz, 1998) from Cox and Alexander's (1995) adult Abbreviated Profile of Hearing Aid Benefit (APHAB).

Some parents write down their observations and activities eagerly and in great detail. Other parents may have difficulty with this, may not enjoy writing, or may feel burdened by this assignment. Let them know it's okay to be brief. The checklist approach or brief log may be easier for these parents. Sometimes parents will return without written information, but will report their observations. It's not so important whether it was written down, but that the assignment gave them structure for observation and involvement and provided the audiologist with important feedback regarding possible adjustments to the hearing aid settings.

Parent Versus Child Responsibilities

Professional opinion varies as to whether parents should be counseled to retain total control over and responsibility for hearing aid care, or whether to also train children to take responsibility as soon as possible for such activities (e.g., asking for and changing batteries and putting in their own earmolds by school age). Elfenbein et al. (1988) reported data to support the inadequacies of even conscientious parental and professional/school monitoring of hearing aids and outlined a program for teaching school-age children to develop hearing aid monitoring skills. The audiologist's professional experience, judgment, and personal style, along with parent and child factors (age, development, and personality), will ultimately determine the approach used, although evidence does support training the child, as well as the parents, to respect and care for the hearing aids to at least some extent.

Keeping the Hearing Aids in Place

Difficulties may arise when fitting hearing aids to very active or accident-prone children, tiny ears, and close-set pinnae. Toupee or hairpiece tape (that is hypo-allergenic and designed for the skin) or surgical tape can be used to secure the hearing aids behind the ears. Fishing line, dental floss, or eyeglass bands can be tied around the earhooks and pinned to the back of the child's shirt or collar. Some companies have designed cute clips that are appealing to children (e.g., Westone Laboratories' Critter Clips or OtoClip for both BTE and ITE hearing aids.) Huggies (Huggie Aids Ltd.) bands are available from a variety of distributors and may also be used to hold hearing aids in place. Keep in mind, too, that well-fitting earmolds will help to keep earmolds and hearing aids in place.

Although ITEs will be less common with younger children, there are circumstances where they may be needed or recommended for younger children or older developmentally delayed children. For these children, loss or damage of the instruments can be deterred by requesting from the hearing aid manufacturer a metal loop on the faceplate, and then attaching fishing line, colored yarn, or dental floss from the loop to the child's clothing.

Counseling the Parents about Feedback Problems

Along with use and care of hearing aids, parents should be informed about the meaning of the presence of hearing aid feedback, including when it's normal and when it's not. Although an in-depth discussion will not be provided here, strategies for reducing problem feedback would include (as appropriate) checking the fit of the earmold (the growing child will require new earmolds frequently), checking for cracks in the earmold or tubing, utilizing a full-shell earmold of soft material with thick or double-walled tubing for severe hearing losses, reducing or eliminating earmold venting, using a longer earmold canal, utilizing an earhook filter, and reducing high-frequency amplification (only as a last resort). Newer multichannel hearing aids and digital signal processing may also be beneficial in managing unwanted feedback.

Counseling Parents Regarding the Limitations of Hearing Aids

Parents should be informed that auditory responsiveness may not be immediate; it may take time for the ears and brain to learn to process new signals. It is also important to explain that hearing aids cannot make hearing "normal." Amplification of sounds, even with advanced signal processing, cannot totally compensate for hearing loss. Auditory dysfunction varies from ear to ear and it is not known exactly how the signal is processed by a given ear. In addition, sound processed through an electronic device is not the same as sound processed through the normal-hearing ear; the amplified signal may not sound "natural." Because hearing aids can amplify unwanted background noise, hearing in noisy environments may be impeded, sometimes severely. Important information can be lost because the hearing aid microphone is not always close to the signal source. Even if it is not known if a given child will be able to process speech information well with his hearing aids, it is important for parents to be aware that hearing aids are not worn solely for speech reception or production; audition for sound awareness to environmental warning sounds and augmentation of speechreading can be important, as well.

FM Systems and Other Assistive Devices

Along with discussion of the limitations of hearing aids, parents must be informed of the benefits of FM, infrared, and induction-loop systems in improving the signal-to-noise ratio by reducing the problems associated with speaker distance, and listening in background noise and reverberation. Although there are many potential applications for FM systems, their importance in the classroom (for children with unilateral *or* bilateral hearing loss) cannot be overemphasized. To this end, hearing aids ordered for children must be compatible with FM devices. Before proposing a specific FM model, it will be helpful to know which FM systems may already be in use in the child's educational program. Other devices and services for telecommunications (closed captioning, TDD/TTY, and relay services) and for alerting or signaling should be discussed as well.

THE CHILD WHO REJECTS AMPLIFICATION

Ruling Out a Hearing Aid/Equipment Problem

After carefully fitting amplification and counseling the parents, it may seem logical to attribute hearing aid rejection to behavioral/psychosocial factors. While this will probably be the case more often than not, a problem with the amplification system itself must be ruled out first. Factors to consider include: amplification exceeding loudness comfort levels (does the child grimace or cover his ears in response to some sounds?); distorted or inadequate signals providing little or no auditory benefit (as, for example, with some severe or profound hearing losses); poorly fitting earmolds such that the volume control setting is reduced to prevent feedback, resulting in insufficient amplification; poorly fitting earmolds causing discomfort; and malfunction of the equipment—even if new. Remind parents how important their observations are in trying to identify these factors. Feedback from teachers and other educational staff can be valuable, as well. If the child is unable to tolerate amplification in certain environments (e.g., very noisy), but does well in others, or if hearing is fluctuating, programmable analog and digital instruments should be considered (not to imply that there are not other good reasons to try programmable and digital instruments).

Hearing Aid Rejection That Is Not Due to Equipment Problems

Just because children reject hearing aids does not mean they are not benefiting from them. Hearing aid rejection is not uncommon and may reflect influences of parental attitudes, rejection of parental authority, peer pressure, or cosmetic concerns. Younger children may attempt to manipulate their parents with fussing, complaining, or even throwing tantrums when the hearing aids are put on. Older children may also use hearing aid rejection to manipulate their parents or to reject authority. A larger issue with adolescents and teenagers is a cosmetic one— looking different and "standing out from the crowd." These factors need to be dealt with early to prevent cosmetics and peer pressure from becoming a negative influence.

Influence of Parental Attitudes, Advocacy, and Discipline

Of prime importance at any age are parental attitudes toward the hearing aids. The child's rejection may be a reflection of attitudes from parents who do not accept amplification. Children quickly pick up on parent attitudes. For example:

- The parents may view the hearing aids as a sign of illness, developmental delay, or weakness—the child's and, by association, the parents'.
- Parents of children who are identified at a later age (e.g., school-age) may not encourage hearing aid use because they don't understand that the child needs to wear hearing aids all the time, not just in school. ("He got along pretty well at home before he got the hearing aids.")
- Parents whose child has a high-frequency hearing loss may not accept their child's need for amplification because the child responds quickly to many environmental sounds, turns around when called, and is using speech and language.

- Although the child with a high-frequency hearing loss may have a "lisp" or other articulation problems, it may be even more difficult for parents to accept the need for hearing aids for the child with a "cookie-bite" hearing loss configuration. Speech and language deficits may not be apparent with this loss, and the child may hear many softer low-frequency and high-frequency sounds well. Because of the valuable information in the mid-frequencies, however, these children will miss the nuances of language and will likely misinterpret things that are said in their environments.
- The parents may feel bothered by or insecure about having to care for the hearing aids and monitor their use, so they may not follow through with encouraging hearing aid use and maintenance.
- The parents may have philosophical beliefs that their child should bear sole responsibility for the use of the hearing aids and, thus, not provide their child with needed guidance and support.

Parents need to advocate for their child, educate others, and be aware of situations where the child may be treated inappropriately (e.g., being teased, stared at, or harassed). On the other hand, low expectations or overprotection of the child may bring on additional teasing and may not allow the child to develop his skills in handling interpersonal relationships and in "growing up." Advocating for the child involves modeling appropriate, natural attitudes toward hearing aids as just another individual variation, and also giving the child tools to handle difficult situations. Children need to trust their parents and be encouraged to share and work through problems. If this is not happening, family counseling may be recommended to give these tools to both the parents and the child.

It is important that both professionals and parents do not discount the child's feelings and use positive reinforcement whenever possible. The child should be comfortable in the audiologist's office and with the audiologist. Explanations directed to the child, along with a little fun and reward, will help build a trusting relationship that will enhance hearing aid use.

With younger children, amplification-enhanced communication should be fun. Putting on the hearing aids and then sitting and being drilled on pronunciation is boring. Reading a book together and talking about it, watching TV, listening to music, talking while having a snack, or playing games with sound in an undemanding environment are fun.

Also, limits should be set and then adhered to (with the realization, as mentioned earlier, that there may be times of stress in which usual routines may be changed, for example, when the child is ill). Children need consistency. Being consistent and setting limits tells children you care and gives them a framework in which to grow and develop. Being consistent means both parents working together and not sending the child mixed messages. It also means that discipline is consistent for *all* children in the family. Setting limits does not mean the child cannot have choices, however. Offering the child choices maintains parental authority while at the same time allows the child to have some control over the situation. Of vital importance in verbal (and nonverbal) expressions of discipline is the distinction between the behavior and the person: the *behavior* is "bad," not the *child.*

Children who are in school or preschool may be assisted in transitioning to use of amplification in the classroom through class orientations or "show and tell." This may be done by the audiologist or by the child (depending on the age) with the assistance of a supportive teacher or other school professional. However, it is wise to talk to the child before any class presentation is done, because some children are mortified by *any* attention that is drawn to them. In these instances, a meeting with the teacher(s) only, or one-to-one ongoing student support and counseling is important.

Cosmetic Concerns or Rejection of Authority

Attempts should be made to determine the reason or reasons for rejection of the hearing aids. This is not always an easy task, and the parents may not be aware that their child just doesn't want to wear one or both hearing aids. The child may complain about the function of one or both of the hearing aids, when it's really an issue of not wanting to wear it/ them. The child may have the parents convinced it is an equipment or comfort problem rather than a cosmetic issue or a rejection of parental authority. Children of middle-school and high-school age don't want to look different; they want to "fit in" and be "cool." At this age, it is not at all uncommon for children to reject hearing aids outright. Input from school personnel may be helpful in identifying factors associated with hearing aid rejection.

If good rapport has been established with adolescents or teenagers, it may be helpful to sit down with them alone. Sometimes they will share their concerns with the audiologist when the parent is not present. Try to get them to talk about themselves: where they've been and how they've coped, how they feel about their world, and what they see happening in the future if various routes are taken. Listening and letting them express their feelings, and validating those feelings, is critical. ("No, it *isn't* fair.") Empathize with them and reinforce positive behavior, then counsel them in a sincere manner as to why amplification is important for their success and well-being. Role-playing may be used to anticipate peer reactions and their responses to them. It's helpful to illustrate the practical impact of amplification, rather than just trying to explain verbally. For example, their performance can be demonstrated in different listening situations with and without hearing aids. They may think they're doing fine, not realizing what they've missed or misinterpreted. A teenage male asking a girl out on a date may be more embarrassed by appearing foolish or ignorant when he responds inappropriately to the girl's answer or questions than if he wore his hearing aids (which she likely knows he wears anyway) and responded appropriately. Telephone use is usually very important to teenagers. Being able to communicate over the phone may be enough of a reinforcement to gain cooperation in using amplification. Never neglect the importance of telephone use when considering amplification options for adolescents and teenagers. This may involve obtaining a stronger hearing aid telecoil and/or a telephone amplifying device. Their amplification system should also allow them to utilize assistive listening devices for group events.

If the issue of hearing aid rejection appears to be not so much a cosmetic issue as a power struggle with the parents or rejection of parental authority, the audiologist may be able to counsel the parents on compromise and offer suggestions for approaching their adolescent or teenager. Some parents will be accepting of this and appreciate the insight; others will not. Refer for professional counseling when appropriate. Rejection of parental authority might be evident in such behaviors as ignoring parent comments or questions, distancing themselves physically from their parents, lack of eye contact with their parents, or using disrespectful language with their parents (in the appointment room or overheard outside the room while waiting or leaving). Rejection of authority may be directed at the audiologist, as well, especially if the audiologist displays a "You have to do this" attitude, rather than one that is encouraging and understanding.

Sometimes contracts between the parents and child, teacher and child, or audiologist and child can be utilized effectively. Offering choices and compromise assists in minimizing authoritativeness. Despite all efforts at explaining how they'll be more "with it" communicatively in social situations, it may be necessary to contract, for example, to wear the hearing aids at school, but not wear them when "hanging out" with their friends. Or, they may be allowed to wear the hearing aids part-time at school if their grades don't drop. If they resist binaural amplification and feel that wearing only one hearing aid is less conspicuous, they may be allowed to wear one instead of two hearing aids if they will wear one consistently. None of these compromises is particularly appealing to the concerned parent or audiologist, and should only be used as last resorts, but if the alternative is total rejection of hearing aids, the child has gained something rather than nothing.

Switching from BTE to ITE hearing aids can also be effective. The disadvantages of ITEs for younger persons (e.g., safety issues for active kids with a hard case inside the ear, frequent recasing as the child grows, incompatibility with assistive listening devices, etc.) must be weighed against the disadvantages of not wearing amplification at all. Older children who reject their BTEs but are happy about wearing ITEs may be more responsible with their use and care. Other obstacles can often be dealt with, as well (e.g., ordering an ITE with a flexible canal and choosing a hearing aid manufacturer that has a recasing/insurance policy, the cost of which may be the same or even less than the cost of new earmolds for BTEs). Ordering hearing aid cases and earmolds with fun colors, or colors to match hair color, may appeal to some children and allow them to "make a statement."

Peer support is often more effective than adult attempts to convince the adolescent or teenager to wear amplification. If possible, try to put teenagers in touch with other teenagers who are hearing impaired or with slightly older mentors who are hearing impaired. Involving a friend may also be helpful. Motivated audiologists, parents, and educators may want to facilitate teen groups and get-togethers. Materials such as *HiP Magazine*, geared for 8- to 14-year-olds with hearing impairment, can enhance a positive self-image in the adolescent or teenager with hearing impairment. Special summer camps for children with hearing loss are also often motivating.

NONCOMPLIANT PARENTS

Understanding and dealing with nonsupportive parents or families may be even more difficult than dealing with the child or teenager who rejects amplification. Ideally the audiologist's thorough preparation and counseling will prevent parental noncompliance, but in the real world, all best efforts may just not be enough. Sometimes it will be clear that the parents are not following through: they do not keep appointments, they verbalize their reluctance to "force" their child to wear the hearing aids, or they state that they don't feel the hearing aids are really helping. However, noncompliance may not be immediately evident. The parents may tell you that all is going well at home and at school and that the hearing aids are working great, yet the child comes to the audiology appointment without the hearing aids on; or the audiologist is told by the parents that all is well, only to find out from the school that the child has not been wearing the hearing aids and/or has not even brought them to school.

The parents must clearly understand the relationship between the child's hearing loss and amplification, and the implications of not amplifying or not following through on appointments and follow-up. As in all phases of counseling, try to find out where they are in their thinking, what they've done or tried, and what they see in the future, with concrete examples of their concerns or reasons for rejecting amplification so that these can be appropriately addressed. This may require probing into family dynamics to gain a better understanding of where the breakdown might be.

All members of a family are affected when one has hearing loss. Spousal tension and conflict may compromise the child's acceptance of and success with amplification, especially if the parents have differing philosophies (where one accepts the diagnosis and/or recommendations but the other does not) or the parents are separated or divorced and are sending the child mixed messages and applying discipline inconsistently. Perhaps the parents are still concerned about the child being mocked by others for wearing amplification. Just because strategies were offered early-on in counseling to cope with reactions or ridicule from others does not mean that these ideas were effectively applied or are even remembered. Much of the information conveyed to parents bears repeating or reviewing. Because the stress of parenting is often compounded by a special needs child—and the addition of hearing aids to an already hectic schedule—parents may need to be reminded to take time out for themselves, both individually and as a couple. They need to be there for each other, and for themselves as individuals, in order to meet their child's needs. A single parent will especially need the support of friends and the extended family.

In addition to parents, other family members may impede the child's acceptance and successful use of amplification. Grandparents can be great sources of support for the family, but they, too, may have difficulty accepting the child's hearing impairment and the need for special intervention, especially if left out of "the loop." Siblings are also an integral part of family dynamics and, as mentioned earlier, are important to the habilitative/rehabilitative process. A child who is hearing impaired may have a positive and educational effect on the sibling. A supportive sibling can lend assistance and encouragement to the child who is hearing impaired at school, at play, and at home. Conversely, a sibling who is not receiving as much attention as the child with hearing loss may feel rejected, insecure, or resentful and may, consciously or unconsciously, undermine the success and well-being of their brother or sister with hearing loss. The hearing impairment should be discussed openly, using language appropriate to the sibling's developmental level. Some problems of family dynamics will likely be beyond the scope of that which the audiologist can address or provide. Again, know when and where to refer.

There will likely be parents who blatantly reject all efforts of the audiologist. In such cases, some professionals advocate threats to turn the parents over to authorities for child abuse or neglect if they do not follow through with amplification. The warning alone often gets their attention. A professional trusted by the family, such as a social worker or religious advisor, or a family friend may be helpful in providing insight and in eliciting cooperation if the audiologist is unsuccessful.

The realization may come that certain parents just cannot be compelled to cooperate. It may be possible to find an educational support person (e.g., a school nurse, school speech-language pathologist, itinerant teacher for the hearing impaired, special education teacher, school counselor, or classroom teacher), who takes a special interest in the child and is willing to keep the hearing aids at school and make sure they are on the student and functioning while the student is at school. Of course, if the school is fortunate enough to have an educational audiologist, she could be an ideal advocate for the child.

DISCREPANCIES IN TEST RESULTS AND DIAGNOSIS

Presenting a diagnosis, test results, and recommendations that differ from those obtained previously from someone else can be particularly challenging. This may involve telling parents who thought their child had normal hearing that he has a hearing loss or, conversely, that the child whom they thought had hearing loss and may already be wearing hearing aids (at probable considerable investment of time, emotion, and cost) does not have hearing loss. The parents may have become adjusted to the fact that their child has normal hearing or is hearing impaired, and now a "can of worms" is opened by changing their reality and their focus. Even if they may have doubted the prior diagnosis, they likely adjusted at some level and may not want to go through the work that this shift in thought and energy may entail. "Why was I told something different?" "Why didn't they see what you are seeing?" "How can you be sure?" "Wouldn't the doctor have known?"

In some cases, the possibility of progressive hearing loss may exist. This cannot be overlooked in counseling the parents regarding intertest differences, especially if some time has elapsed between evaluations. Test results may also be interpreted differently once more information is obtained to define the results better, especially for a child who is, or has been, difficult to test.

It may not necessarily be possible to explain the prior results and diagnosis in the context of the present findings, even if it appears that the diagnosis was incorrect, nor is it necessarily desirable to try to do so. Although it may be helpful to address factors that may have influenced the prior test results, such as false positives, doing so in a professional manner does not have to involve criticizing or accusing another professional. As tempting as it is to lay blame on another person in order to persuade the parent to believe current findings, it does not serve the profession well or necessarily take into account everything that may have transpired or difficulties *anyone* may encounter at one time or another (e.g., the possibility of progressive hearing loss or even of "making a mistake"). It does seem responsible whenever possible, however, to share the results with the other professional, in a tactful way, so that it becomes a learning experience.

That said, it is advisable to focus instead on the present results and the reasons they are believed to be an actual representation of the child's current auditory function. This may mean demonstrating further. For example, in counseling parents of children who display functional hearing loss, there can be an explanation and demonstration of the inconsistencies of obtaining a normal speech reception threshold and perfect word recognition scores at soft conversational levels in the presence of elevated pure-tone responses. An inquiry into and discussion of factors that may have precipitated the child's need to malinger— what the child hoped to gain—can be helpful to parents in accepting the test results and guiding them toward further intervention (removal of hearing aids if they had been placed, counseling, etc.), if indicated.

Perhaps even more difficult, however, may be explaining to the parents that their child needs hearing aids when they had been told previously that "everything is fine." The inherent difficulties often associated with testing children both behaviorally and nonbehaviorally (depending on development level, cooperation, activity level and restlessness, for example), and the limitations of the range of testing that may be provided in one clinic versus another, should be explained to the parents. Use and explanation of nonbehavioral tests, including otoacoustic emissions, auditory brainstem response testing, and acoustic reflexes, assist the audiologist in confirming the diagnosis and assist the parents in accepting the diagnosis. Again, demonstration can be invaluable. Parents involved in the testing process are more likely to become aware of what their child is and is not responding to. It may also be beneficial, if possible, to have a teacher or other professional (such as the child's speech-language pathologist) present to "witness" the testing process and results. Because the parents did not want to "hear" this new diagnosis, they may reject the current audiologist, and the parent-professional relationship may become strained. If this is not quickly resolved, it may be advisable for the child and parents to proceed with amplification with another audiologist so that the child's chance for success is not compromised.

COUNSELING PARENTS WHO ARE DEAF

Different issues arise when the audiologist is working with parents who are deaf. In all likelihood, deaf parents will be prepared to have deaf children whom they will raise in the Deaf Culture; the audiologist may be minimally involved. Some may question if it is even appropriate for audiologists to try to provide deaf parents of deaf children with counseling. However, some deaf parents may choose to raise their hard-of-hearing or deaf children bilingually (ASL and English) and biculturally (within the hearing world and within the Deaf Culture). Knowledge of, sensitivity to, and respect for the Deaf Culture in dealing with deaf parents is imperative. If deaf parents do not want to amplify their hard-of-hearing child because they are a part of the deaf community (particularly if the child is hearing impaired but not deaf), the question may arise as to whether this constitutes neglect of their child. Or, should the parents' decision be respected as long as the child develops a communication system to use within that family and culture? The answers (if there are any) certainly cannot be provided here, but it seems reasonable to be prepared (utilizing a proficient interpreter) to evaluate the children of deaf parents, to explain and discuss the results and implications of the hearing loss, whatever the degree, and to provide intervention, resources, follow-up, and support if requested and needed.

CONCLUSIONS

Parent support and involvement may affect a child's success with amplification as much, if not more, than the particular amplification system used, the educational approach, the audiologist, or the particular child. To be their child's best advocate, parents need to have a clear understanding of their child, their options for intervention, and their child's hearing loss and amplification system, and then be guided to be, not only active participants, but leaders in decision making throughout their child's habilitative/rehabilitative process. Parents should be counseled that the intervention process is not stagnant, but constantly evolving; changes will be made throughout the child's growth and development as new information and experiences are assimilated.

We as audiologists owe it to the children we serve, their parents, and ourselves to become the best professionals we can by staying current in the field, understanding our limitations by making appropriate referrals when necessary, and maintaining (and conveying) realistic expectations of amplification. Parents must feel confident in the audiologist as their professional expert, and confident in themselves as the parent expert of their child. No one audiologist can meet all the needs of all of his or her patients or even any one child or family; but strengthening of counseling and interpersonal skills will facilitate the building of a cooperative working relationship with the parents, who ultimately enable the successful amplification of their children with hearing impairment.

REFERENCES

Arnos, K. S., Downs, K., Israel, J. I., & Cunningham, M. (1989, July/August). Genetics and hearing impairment: What is genetic counseling? *Shhh*, pp. 10–13.

Cox, R. M., & Alexander, G. C. (1995). The abbreviated profile of hearing aid benefit. *Ear and Hearing, 16*, 176–183.

Diefendorf, A. O., Chaplin, R. G., Kessler, K. S., Miller, S. M., Miyamoto, R. T., Myres, W. A., Pope, M. L., Reitz, P. S., Renshaw, J. J., Steck, J. T., & Wagner, M. L. (1990). Follow-up and intervention: Completing the process. *Seminars in Hearing, 11*, 393–407.

Elfenbein, J. L., Bentler, R. A., Davis, J. M., & Niebuhr, D. P. (1988). Status of school children's hearing aids relative to monitoring practices. *Ear and Hearing, 9*, 212–217.

Johnson, C. D. (1997). Understanding and advising parents and families. *The Hearing Review, 18*–20.

Kopun, J. G., & Stelmachowicz, P. G. (1998). Perceived communication difficulties of children with hearing loss. *American Journal of Audiology, 7*, 30–38.

Luterman, D. M. (1985). The denial mechanism. *Ear and Hearing, 6*, 57–58.

Rushmer, N. (1994). Supporting families of hearing-impaired infants and toddlers. *Seminars in Hearing, 15*, 160–172.

Stelmachowicz, P. G., Larson, L. L., Johnson, D. E., & Moeller, M. P. (1985). Clinical model for the audiological management of hearing-impaired children. *Seminars in Hearing, 6*, 223–237.

APPENDIX 9–A

Support Materials for Parents and Families

The following materials may be helpful to parents and families. The information may be assembled in a parent notebook of resources or may be given to the parents separately at times deemed appropriate by the audiologist. Not all materials listed may be appropriate for all parents.

- **Diagrams and audiometric information:** explanations of different hearing loss types, diagram of the ear, sample audiogram, a copy of the child's audiogram, loudness levels of various environmental sounds, the "speech banana," speech sounds plotted on the audiogram.
- **Options in education:** including written information on auditory/ oral, cued speech, sign language, total communication, and various program combination options, as well as local programs or contacts. (See Organizations in Appendix 9–C, some of which target different approaches.)
- **Local and national organizations listing:** contact information including addresses, phone numbers, web sites, and e-mail addresses. (See Appendix 9–C for national listings.)
- **Financial resources:** contact information for local, county, state, and national resources for financial assistance for amplification and education. (See listings in Appendix 9–C, which include financial resources.)
- **Internet/Web sites:** this information may be listed separately or included in other listings such as local and national resource listings, and may also include newsgroups and parent support groups. (See Organizations list in Appendix 9–C for some web site information.)
- **Communication strategies:** for example, "Help Me Talk: A Parent's Guide to Speech and Language Stimulation Techniques for Children 1 to 3 Years," (1993), available from Pi Communication Materials, P.O. Box 2508, Glen Allen, VA 23058, (800) 254-0444. Also check with local speech-language pathologists for more information.
- **Informational handouts:** such as the Educational Audiology Association's Hearing Loss Counseling Pads with tear-off sheets with the implications of various degrees of hearing loss (available from the Educational Audiology Association—see listing in Appendix 9–C); hearing health care tips, including information on hearing protection devices and noise damage fact sheets, such as those available from the New York League for the Hard of Hearing (see listing in Appendix 9–C); information on otitis media; and tips for teachers.

- **Books and pamphlets:** a listing or "lending library" of favorite materials. Also see suggested readings in Appendix 9–B.
- **Hearing aids and their use and care:** materials personally designed and/or those provided by hearing instrument manufacturers, especially those specifically directed to children and parents.
- **Child materials:** activity kits, materials, and web sites, such as those sponsored by some hearing instrument manufacturers and by Sertoma International; books (e.g., *Patrick Gets Hearing Aids*, 1994, M.C. Riski & N. Klakow, Naperville, IL: Phonak) or subscriptions, such as *HiP Magazine* for adolescents 8–14 years old with hearing impairment. (See *HiP Magazine* listing in Appendix 9–C.)
- **Video and audio tapes:** such as, *Beginnings* (a parent-education tape from the organization Beginnings for Parents of Hearing-Impaired Children, Inc., listed in Appendix 9–C); *My Child is Deaf, What Do I Do Now?* (available from the House Ear Institute, listed in Appendix 9–C); *Understanding Hearing Loss* (a 17-minute video simulating hearing loss, demonstrating hearing loss with no visual cues, and demonstrating communication in noise, from Films for the Humanities, Inc., Princeton, 1993); and *Families with Deaf Children: Discovering Your Needs, Exploring Your Choices* and *Families with Hard-of-Hearing Children: What if Your Child Has a Hearing Loss?* (produced by Boys Town National Research Hospital, listed in Appendix 9–C).
- **Parent hearing aid care kit:** items to include a listening stethoscope; battery tester; dri-aid jar/kit; forced-air blower; cleaning tools (wax loop and brush); extra batteries; earmold lubricant, if necessary; and earmold sanitizer, if necessary.
- **Information on pertinent legislation and regulations, including:**

Education for All Children With Disabilities

PL (Public Law) 94-142: The Education for All Handicapped Children Act (1975).
Requires that all handicapped children ages 5–21 years old receive a free and appropriate public education at public expense. Includes the right of parents to be involved in making decisions about their child.

PL 99-457 (1986).
Amendment to PL 94-142 which expands the ages of PL 94-142 and mandates free and appropriate services for all infants and toddlers. Title II: 3–5 years old; Title I, Part H: 0 through 2 years old.

PL 101-476 (1990): Individuals with Disabilities Education Act (IDEA)
Amendments which reauthorized and expanded Part B of PL 94-142.

PL 102-119 IDEA Amendments (1991).

PL 105-17 (H.R. 5, S. 717) IDEA Amendments (1997).

Signed into law June 4, 1997, approval in 1998 pending actual regulations that will implement the law.

- *Part A: General Provisions* (School Age Program).
- *Part B: Assistance for Education of All Children with Disabilities* (School Age Program).
- *Part C: Infants and Toddlers with Disabilites* (Formerly Part H).
- *Part D: National Activities to Improve Education of Children with Disabilities* (Six programs: State Improvement Grants; Research and Innovation; Personnel Preparation; Studies and Evaluations; Coordinated Technical Assistance/Information Dissemination, including parent training and information centers; and Technology Development, Demonstration, and Utilization/Educational Media Service).

Rehabilitation Act of 1973 (PL 93-112)
Recent reauthorization passed as part of a larger job training consolidation bill signed into law on August 7, 1998 by President Clinton. The Rehabilitation Act provides a framework to help Americans with disabilities pursue meaningful careers through vocational training and rehabilitation.

Section 504 of the Rehabilitation Act
Prevents recipients of federal financial assistance from discriminating on the basis of disability in their programs or activities. Discrimination against students on the basis of handicap is prohibited in educational programs or activities, including elementary and secondary as well as post-secondary schools. *Federal Register, 42,* May 4, 1977.

Americans with Disabilities Act (ADA) of 1990 (PL 101-336)
This Act gives civil rights protection to persons with disabilities and guarantees equal opportunity for individuals with disabilities in employment (Title I), transportation (Title II), state and local government services (Title II), privately owned public accommodations (Title III), and telecommunications (Title IV). Title V contains miscellaneous standards and compliance details. This Act extends the provisions of the Rehabilitation Act of 1973 throughout both public and private sectors regardless of funding sources.

Miscellaneous Legislated Rules and Agency Regulations

Federal
- *Food and Drug Administration (FDA).* The FDA *Code of Federal Regulations* (CFR) is a codification of rules published in the *Federal Register*

by executive departments and agencies of the federal government. The Rules and Regulations for hearing aid device labeling and conditions of sale in the *Federal Register,* Vol. 42, No. 31, February 15, 1977 (21 CFR Parts 801.420 and .421) established regulations regarding hearing aids, which were last revised as of April 1, 1998. These regulations include:

Hearing aid devices: Professional and patient labeling (801.420):
(a) definitions ("hearing aid," "ear specialist," "dispenser," "audiologist," "sale or purchase," "used hearing aid"); (b) label requirements for hearing aids; and (c) The User Instructional Booklet requirements to accompany each hearing aid, including technical data which may be in the User Booklet or in separate labeling that accompanies the hearing aid.

Hearing aid devices: Conditions for sale (801.421):
(a) medical evaluation requirements, including a medical evaluation and signed medical clearance within the preceding six months, or a signed waiver to the medical evaluation requirements (with particular waiver requirements specified) if the prospective hearing user is 18 years old or older; (b) opportunity to review the User Instructional Brochure prior to signing a waiver; (c) requirements for availability of a User Instructional Brochure; (d) record-keeping requirements for retaining the medical clearance or waiver for three years after dispensing a hearing aid); and (e) exemptions for "group auditory trainers."

■ *Social Security Administration (SSA).* See contact information in Appendix 9–C. Benefits that may be pertinent to children include:

Supplemental Security Income (SSI). Federal cash assistance program for children and adults with significant disabilities. Provides monthly payments for needy children under 18 who have a severe disability or chronic illness. The federal government pays a basic rate and some states add to that amount. Generally people who get SSI also qualify for Medicaid, food stamps, and other assistance. (SSI benefits are not based on past earnings.)

Social Security Disability Benefits. Payable at any age to people who have enough Social Security credits and who have a severe physical or mental impairment that is expected to prevent them from working for a year or more, or who have a condition that is expected to result in death.

Social Security Family Benefits. Spouses (under some conditions) and unmarried children under age 18 (or under 19 but still in school, or older but disabled) might receive benefits if a parent is eligible for retirement or disability benefits.

Social Security Survivor Benefits. Spouses (under some conditions) and unmarried children under age 18 (or under 19 but still in school, or older but disabled) might receive benefits if a parent dies and the parent earned enough Social Security credits while working.

State or Local

- *Professional licenses or registration.* See listing in Appendix 9–C for the National Council of State Boards of Examiners for Speech-Language Pathology and Audiology. Also see the American Speech-Language-Hearing Association web site for listings of state regulatory agencies for hearing aid dispensers and for speech-language pathologists and audiologists.
- *Requirements for hearing aid trial periods.*
- *Medicaid.* Pays for health care for eligible persons who are aged, disabled, pregnant, or refugees, and who meet income and poverty guidelines.
- *State offices of education and educational programs for the hearing impaired.* See U. S. Department of Education listings in Appendix 9–C.
- *Other state or local funding for medical, hearing aid, or intervention services for children with special needs.*

Further information and resources regarding legislation and regulations can be found in the Suggested Readings and Organizations listings of Appendixes 9–B and 9–C. Further state and local information is often included in local telephone books. The listing in Appendix 9–C for the National Information Center for Children and Youth with Disabilities provides individual state resources lists.

APPENDIX 9–B

Suggested Readings for Parents and/or Professionals

Books

Bitter, G. (1978). *Parents in action.* Washington, DC: Alexander Graham Bell Association for the Deaf. [Experiences of parents raising children who are hearing impaired.]

Bull, T. H. (Ed.). (1998). *On the edge of deaf culture: Hearing children/deaf parents annotated bibliography.* Alexandria, VA: Deaf Family Research Press.

Featherstone, H. (1981). *A difference in the family: Living with a disabled child.* New York: Penguin Books. [A parent's experience in dealing with her child's severe disabilities.]

Ferris, C. (1980). *A hug just isn't enough.* Washington, DC: Gallaudet University. [Experiences of parents of children who are hearing-impaired.]

Ferris, M. T. (1994). *Bright silence: Raising hearing-impaired children.* Neenah, WI: Bright Silence Press.

Harris, G. (1983). *Broken ears, wounded hearts.* Washington, DC: Gallaudet University. [Personal experience of growing up with a deaf girl.]

Johnson, C. D., Benson, P. V., & Seaton, J. B. (1997). *Educational Audiology Handbook.* San Diego: Singular Publishing Group, Inc. [Includes family relationships and parent resources, in addition to educational audiology practices, amplification, needs assessment, governmental policies, performance measures, and extensive appendixes.]

Luterman, D. M. (1979). *Counseling parents of hearing-impaired children.* Boston: Little, Brown and Co.

Luterman, D. M. (1991). *When your child is deaf: A guide for parents.* Parkton, MD: York Press.

Luterman, D. M. (1996). *Counseling persons with communication disorders and their families* (3rd ed.). Austin, TX: Pro-Ed.

Maxon, A. B., & Brackett, D. (1992). *The hearing-impaired child: Infancy through high school years.* Stoneham, MA: Andover Medical Publishers, Inc. [Auditory, speech, language, and educational management strategies for treating hearing loss of all degrees for all ages of children.]

Meyer, D. J., Vadasy, P. F., & Fewell, R. R. (1996). *Living with a brother or sister with special needs: A book for sibs* (2nd ed.). Seattle: University of Washington Press.

Peterson, J. (1977). *I have a sister—My sister is deaf.* New York: Harper & Row.

Powell, T., & Gallagher, P. A. (1993). *Brothers and sisters: A special part of exceptional families* (2nd ed.). Baltimore: Paul H. Brookes.

Roeser, R. J., & Downs, M. P. (1995). *Auditory disorders in school children: The law, identification, remediation* (3rd ed.). New York: Thieme Medical Publishers, Inc.

Rousch, J., & Matkin, N. D. (Eds.). (1994). *Infants and toddlers with hearing loss: Family centered assessment and intervention.* Parkton, MD: York Press.

Schwartz, S. (Ed.). (1996). *Choices in deafness: A parent's guide to communication options* (2nd ed.). Bethesda, MD: Woodbine House. [Includes professional and parental viewpoints and experiences with oral, cued speech, and total communication approaches, as well as medical and resource information.]

Tucker, B. P. (1997). *IDEA advocacy for children who are deaf or hard-of-hearing: A question and answer book for parents and professionals.* San Diego: Singular Publishing Group, Inc.

Articles/Pamphlets/Booklets

Adkins, D. V. (1987). *Siblings of the hearing-impaired: Perspectives for parents.* Reprint #87-0. Washington, DC: Alexander Graham Bell Association for the Deaf.

Alexander Graham Bell Association for the Deaf. *Parent Packet.* Washington, DC: Author. [Compilation of articles and pamphlets for parents about children with hearing loss. Available for birth to 5 years old, 6–12 years old, and teenagers at $10 per packet.]

Arnos, K. S., Downs, K., Israel, J. I., & Cunningham, M. (1989, July/August). Genetics and hearing impairment: What is genetic counseling? *Shhh,* pp. 10–13.

Diefendorf, A. O., Chaplin, R. G., Kessler, K. S., Miller, S. M., Miyamoto, R. T., Myres, W. A., Pope, M. L., Reitz, P. S., Renshaw, J. J., Steck, J. T., & Wagner, M. L. (1990). Follow-up and intervention: Completing the process. *Seminars in Hearing, 11*(4), 393–407. [Follow-up after early assessment of hearing loss.]

Eichten, P. I. (1993). *Help me talk: A parent's guide to speech and language stimulation techniques for children 1 to 3 years.* Glen Allen, VA: Pi Communications.

Elfenbein, J. L., Bentler, R. A., Davis, J. M., & Niebuhr, D. P. (1988). Status of school children's hearing aids relative to monitoring practices. *Ear and Hearing, 9*(4), 212–217.

Hasenstab, M. S. (Guest Ed.). (1994). Early intervention for infants with hearing impairment. *Seminars in Hearing, 15*(2).

Kopun, J. G., & Stelmachowicz, P. G. (1998). Perceived communication difficulties of children with hearing loss. *American Journal of Audiology, 7,* 30–38.

Luterman, D. M. (1985). The denial mechanism. *Ear and Hearing, 6*(1), 57–58.

Luterman, D. M. (1990, April). Audiological counseling and the diagnostic process. *Asha,* pp. 35–37.

Murphy, A. T. (1979). *The families of hearing-impaired children.* Washington, DC: Alexander Graham Bell Association for the Deaf. [A group of papers in a special issue of *The Volta Review* regarding the impact of hearing impairment on the family.]

National Information Center on Deafness. (1991). *Growing together: Information for parents of deaf and hard of hearing children.* Washington, DC: Author. [Parent booklet available for $8.00 plus shipping.]

Rushmer, N. (1994). Supporting families of hearing-impaired infants and toddlers. *Seminars in Hearing, 15,* 160–172.

Smith, P. M. (1997). You are not alone: For parents when they learn that their child has a disability. *NICHCY News Digest, 20,* February, 2–5. [A parent of a child with multiple disabilities reviews common parent reactions and ways to help the parents through this difficult period.]

Tucker, B. P. (1994). Legal rights of hearing-impaired persons under the Americans with Disabilities Act and related federal laws. *Seminars in Hearing, 13,* 230–242.

U. S. Department of Education. Reprints and publications available by writing to:
United State Department of Education
Office for Civil Rights
Customer Service Team
330 C St. SW
Washington, DC 20202

■ *The Americans With Disabilities Act* (1991). Washington, DC: Department of Justice. [Contains a brief overview of the ADA and lists contact information for the Department of Justice.]

■ *Student placement in elementary and secondary schools and Section 504 and Title II of the Americans with Disabilities Act.* (1996). Washington, DC: Office of Civil Rights. [Describes the Education of the Handicapped Act, now IDEA, which provides federal financial assistance to states to ensure that each child who has a disability receives a free and appropriate education.]

■ *Federal Regulation, May 9, 1980, for Section 504 Regulation of the Rehabilitation Act of 1973 with December 1990 Amendment. A Federal Register* reprint. [Nondiscrimination on the basis of disability in education programs and activities receiving or benefiting from federal financial assistance.]

■ *Federal Regulation, May 9, 1980, for the Title IV Regulation of the Civil Rights Act of 1964. A Federal Register* reprint. [Nondiscrimination on the basis of race, color, or national origin in educational programs and activities receiving or benefiting from federal financial assistance.]

APPENDIX 9–C

Organizations with Information and/or Services for Children with Hearing Loss

Alexander Graham Bell Association for the Deaf, Inc.
3417 Volta Place, NW
Washington, DC 20007-2778
202-337-5220 (Voice/TDD)
agbell2@aol.com (E-mail)
www.agbell.org (Web site)

Nonprofit membership association that promotes public understanding and early detection of hearing loss; educational, vocational, and social opportunities for persons who are hearing impaired (including scholarships); encourages people with hearing impairment to communicate by developing maximum use of residual hearing, speechreading, and speech and language skills; and collaborates on research relating to auditory/verbal communication. A variety of publications is available.

American Academy of Audiology (AAA)
8201 Greensboro Dr., Suite 300
McLean, VA 22102
800-AAA-2336
703-610-9022
703-610-9005 (Fax)
www.audiology.org (Web site)

Professional organization for audiologists, dedicated to providing quality hearing care to the public by enhancing the ability of its members to achieve career and practice objectives through professional development, education, research, and increased public awareness of hearing disorders and audiological services. Informational brochures and referral information are available to consumers and professionals.

American Academy of Otolaryngology—Head and Neck Surgery (AAO-HNS)
One Prince St.
Alexandria, VA 22314-3357
703-836-4444 (Voice)
703-519-1585 (TDD)
703-683-5100 (Fax)
entnews@aol.com (E-mail)
www.entnet.org (Web site)

Information about medicine related to the ear, nose, and throat or head and neck surgery. Pamphlets regarding ear problems, and referrals to physicians are available.

American Hearing Research Foundation
55 East Washington St., Suite 2022
Chicago, IL 60602
312-726-9670

Provides support and grants for medical and educational research into causes, prevention, and cures of hearing loss and balance problems.

American Society for Deaf Children (ASDC)
1820 Tribute Rd., Suite A
Sacramento, CA 95815
800-942-ASDC (Voice/TDD Parent Hotline)
916-641-6084 (Voice/TDD)
916-641-6085 (Fax)
ASDC1@aol.com (E-mail)
www.deafchildren.org (Web site)

International organization of families and professionals committed to educating, empowering, and supporting parents to create opportunities for their children who are deaf or hard of hearing. Promotes a positive attitude toward signing and deaf culture.

American Speech-Language-Hearing Association (ASHA)
10801 Rockville Pike
Rockville, MD 28052-3279
800-498-2071
301-897-5700 (Voice)
301-897-0157 (TDD)
301-571-0457 (Fax)
www.asha.org (Web site)

Professional organization for audiologists and speech-language pathologists dedicated to promoting high-quality services for professionals in speech-language pathology, audiology, and speech and hearing science, and to advocating for people with communication disabilities. A variety of pamphlets and referral information are available to consumers and professionals. The web site includes a listing of state regulatory agencies for hearing aid dispensing and for speech-language pathology and audiology.

Americans with Disabilities Act (ADA) Information Line
United States Department of Justice
800-514-0301 (Voice)
800-514-0383 (TDD)
www.usdoj.gov/crt/ada/infoline.htm (Web site)
ADA Regulations and Technical Assistance Materials/Publications
www.usdoj.gov/crt/ada/publicat.htm (Web site)

AT & T Relay
745 Route 202/206
Bridgewater, NJ 08807
908-231-6081 (TDD)

Auditory-Verbal International, Inc.
2121 Eisenhower Ave., Suite 402
Alexandria, VA 22314
703-739-1049 (Voice)
703-739-0874 (TDD)
703-739-0395 (Fax)
www.auditory-verbal.org (Web site)

Private, nonprofit organization dedicated to promoting listening and speaking as a way of life for children who are deaf or hard of hearing by using their residual hearing, hearing aids, and cochlear implants. Its goals include heightening public awareness of the Auditory-Verbal approach and ensuring certification standards for Auditory-Verbal clinicians and teachers. AVI trains and certifies therapists in the Auditory-Verbal approach in Canada, North America, and some international sites.

Beginnings for Parents of Hearing-Impaired Children, Inc.
North Carolina Council for the Hearing Impaired
3900 Barrett Dr., Suite 100
Raleigh, NC 27609
800-541-4327

Produces materials to help families make choices about communication methods.

Better Hearing Institute (BHI)
5021-B Backlick Rd.
Annandale, VA 22003-6058
800-EAR-WELL (Voice/TDD Hearing Help Line)
888-432-7435 (BHI Office)
703-642-0580 (Voice/TDD)
703-750-9302 (Fax)
mail@betterhearing.org (E-mail)
www.betterhearing.org (Web site)

Nonprofit educational organization that implements national public information programs on hearing loss and available help for hearing loss through medicine, surgery, amplification, and other rehabilitation. Brochures and information are available on hearing loss, tinnitus, and hearing aids, as well as a directory of hearing care providers (audiologists, hearing instrument specialists, and otolaryngologists).

Boys Town National Research Hospital (BTNRH)
555 N. 30th St.
Omaha, NE 68131
402-498-6511 (Voice)
402-498-6543 (TDD)
402-498-6638 (Fax)
www.boystown.org (Web site)

Center for research, diagnosis, and treatment of patients with ear disease, hearing and balance disorders, cleft lip and palate, and speech-language problems. Includes programs such as Parent/Child Workshops, Center for Childhood Deafness, Registry for Hereditary Hearing Loss, Center for Hearing Research, and Center for Abused Handicapped.

Canine Companions for Independence (CCI)
National Headquarters
P.O. Box 446 (2965 Dutton Ave.)
Santa Rosa, CA 95402-0446
800-572-2275 (Voice/TDD)
707-577-1700 (Voice)
707-577-1756 (TDD)
707-577-1711 (Fax)
www.caninecompanions.org (Web site)

Nonprofit organization that provides highly trained assistance dogs to people with disabilities and to professional caregivers providing pet assistance therapy. Assistance dogs are matched to individuals as: Service Dogs, Hearing Dogs, Assisted Service (Social) Dogs, and Facility (Pet Therapy) Dogs. CCI provides continuing support for these teams to ensure success.

Cochlear Implant Club International
5335 Wisconsin Ave., NW, Suite 440
Washington, DC 20015-2003
202-895-2781 (Voice/TDD)
202-895-2782 (Fax)
webmaster@cici.org (E-mail)
www.cici.org (Web site)

Nonprofit organization which provides information and support to cochlear implant users and their families, professionals, and the general public.

Council for Exceptional Children
1920 Association Dr.
Reston, VA 20191
800-328-0272
703-620-3660 (Voice/TDD)

Legislation, development of professional standards, scholarships, and educational information and materials (ERIC Clearinghouse on Disabilities and Gifted Education) to promote education of handicapped and gifted children.

Deafness Research Foundation (DRF)
575 5th Ave., 11th Floor
New York, NY 10017
800-535-DEAF (Voice/TDD)
212-599-0027 (Voice/TDD)
212-599-0039 (Fax)
drf@drf.org (E-mail)
www.drf.org (Web site)

Voluntary health organization that provides research grants related to causes, treatment, and prevention of deafness and all ear disorders. Also provides information and referral services.

Delta Society National Service Dog Center (NSDC)
289 Perimeter Rd. East
Renton, WA 98055
800-869-6898 (Voice)
206-235-1076 (Fax)
deltasociety@cis.compuserve.com (E-mail)
www.deltasociety.org (Web site)

Assists consumers of all ages in locating service dogs or trainers for service dogs. Provides advocacy for persons with service dogs; education to the public regarding service dog issues; information about the selection, training, stewardship, and roles of service animals; referral to service animal training programs and related resources; research assistance through their Resource Library and network of professional experts.

Dogs for the Deaf, Inc.
10175 Wheeler Rd.
Central Point, OR 97502
800-990-DOGS
541-826-9220 (Voice/TDD)
541-826-6696 (Fax)
info@dogsforthedeaf.org (E-mail)
www.dogsforthedeaf.org (Web site)

Nonprofit organization that rescues dogs from animal shelters, trains, and places them with persons who are hearing impaired throughout the United States and Canada at no charge to the recipient. Novice dogs (trained to respond to about 3 sounds) are placed with children as young as 10 years old, home-hearing dogs (trained to respond to up to 7 sounds) are placed with persons who are at least 14 years old, and certified hearing dogs (with public access) are placed with persons with hearing loss who are at least 18 years old.

The Ear Foundation
Baptist Hospital
1817 Patterson St.
Nashville, TN 37203
800-545-HEAR (Voice/TDD)
615-329-7809 (Voice/TDD)
earfound@theearfound.org (E-mail)
www.theearfound.org (Web site)

National nonprofit organization which exists to educate the public and medical profession in matters of hearing loss and ear disease, and to sponsor basic clinical research into hearing and balance disorders. Offers continuing medical education programs, scholarships for the hearing-impaired, educational programs for children, and international outreach programs.

Ear of the Lion Hearing Foundation
2337 Technology Parkway, Suite G
Hollister, CA 95023-2544
800-327-8077
408-634-1351
408-634-1363 (Fax)
eolfoundat@aol.com

A nonprofit foundation formed by the Lion's Clubs of California-Nevada. Its purpose is to provide medical care related to hearing for low-income persons who are not eligible for any government assisted programs. The Hearing Foundation provides hearing aids, medical care, and additional support for citizens who are hearing impaired; financial support for treatment and prevention of deafness; and educational programs on hearing and hearing conservation. Donated, reconditioned, and recased hearing aids are loaned (permanently, if necessary) to low-income persons at $75 per hearing aid. Hearing professionals (audiologists or dispensers) donate their time or are paid $50 by the Lion's Foundation. Interested persons must apply and qualify financially, then are referred by the Foundation to a local resource. Currently services from this chapter are available only in California and Nevada.

Educational Audiology Association
4319 Ehrlich Rd.
Tampa, Florida 33624
800-460-7EAA
813-968-3597 (Fax)
www.edaud.org (Web site)

Membership organization of audiologists who work in the schools or provide services to pre-school and school-age children for educational purposes. A variety of professional materials and publications are available to assist audiologists in providing a full range of appropriate audiological services to children in educational environments.

Gallaudet University
800 Florida Ave., NE
Washington, DC 20002-3695
800-672-6720
202-651-5000 (Voice/TDD)
www.gallaudet.edu (Web site)

A liberal arts university for deaf and hearing persons. (The world's only 4-year liberal arts university for deaf or hard of hearing persons.) Provides more than 50 undergraduate and graduate degree programs and numerous continuing education and summer courses. Disseminates information through the Gallaudet Bookstore, Gallaudet University Press, Gallaudet Research Institute, Pre-College National Missions Programs, College for Continuing Education, and the National Information Center on Deafness (NICD). [Also see listing for NICD.]

Health Resource Center
One Dupont Circle, NW, Suite 800
Washington, DC 20036-1193
800-544-3284

Information on financial aid for students with disabilities.

Hear Now
9745 E. Hampden Ave., Suite 300
Denver, CO 80231-4923
800-648-HEAR (Voice/TDD)
303-695-7797 (Voice/TDD)
303-695-7789 (Fax)
127737.1272@compuserve.com (E-mail)
www.leisurelan.com/hearnow (Web site)

National bank of new and refurbished used hearing aids that are dispensed through approved local hearing health care professionals (who agree to fit the aids at no charge) if financial eligibility criteria are met. Includes financial assistance for cochlear implants by coordinating philanthropic efforts of implant manufacturers, implant teams, and local fundraising leaders.

Hearing Education and Awareness for Rockers (H.E.A.R.)
Mailing address:
P.O. Box 460847
San Francisco, CA 94146
H.E.A.R. Office:
University of California-San Francisco Center on Deafness
3333 California St., Suite 10
San Francisco, CA 94118
415-441-9081 (Voice)
415-476-7600 (TDD)
415-552-4296 (Fax)
415-773-9590 (24-hr. National Information Hotline)
hear@hearnet.com (E-mail)
www.hearnet.com (Web site)

Nonprofit organization founded by musicians and physicians for musicians, music lovers, and other music professionals. Offers information about dangers of repeated exposure to excessive noise levels, hearing protection, ear monitor systems, testing, hearing loss, and tinnitus; public awareness campaigns and public service announcements; referral and support network; and free hearing clinic program.

Hearing Rehabilitation Foundation
35 Medford St.
Somerville, MA 02143
617-628-4537
HeaRF@aol.com (E-mail)

Small nonprofit foundation dedicated to promoting speech communication training for children and adults with profound hearing loss. Educational seminars and workshops are provided about the Foundation's speech training program, which is part of a bilingual-bicultural-bimodal model. Some hearing-impaired people are seen at the Foundation for direct services.

The HIKE Fund, Inc. (Hearing Impaired Kids Endowment Fund)
c/o International Center for Job's Daughters
233 W. 6th St.
Papillion, NE 68046-2210
401-592-7987
402-592-2177 (Fax)
sgc@iojd.org (E-mail)

Financial assistance for hearing aids, FMs, closed caption devices, tactile aids, alerting systems, and specialized sports equipment (but not cochlear implants) for children 0–20 years with financial need.

HiP Magazine, Inc.
1563 Solano Ave., #137
Berkeley, CA 94707
510-848-9650 (Voice)
510-848-9639 (Fax)

Informational, educational, and activity-oriented magazine for adolescents (8–14 years old) with hearing impairment.

House Ear Institute
2100 W. 3rd St.
Los Angeles, CA 90057
213-483-4431 (Voice)
213-484-2642 (TDD)
213-483-8789 (Fax)
webmaster@hei.org (E-mail)
www.hei.org (Web site)
Lead Line:
800-287-4763 (Voice/TDD in California)
800-352-8888 (Voice/TDD in all other states)
CARE Center:
213-353-7005 (Voice)
213-483-2226 (TDD)
213-483-3716 (Fax)

Private, nonprofit organization which provides services, education, and research into ear disorders. The Lead Line provides a nationwide information and referral service. It assists families in making confident and well-informed decisions concerning the rearing and education of their deaf and hard of hearing children.

The Children's Auditory Research and Evaluation (CARE) Center offers pediatric otologic and audiologic evaluation and treatment, rehabilitation, hearing aid dispensing, and cochlear implant services. Outreach programs focus on families with children who are hearing impaired.

International Hearing Dog, Inc.
5901 East 89th Ave.
Henderson, CO 80640
303-287-3277 (Voice/TDD)
ihdi@aol.com (E-mail)

Hearing dogs for persons with hearing loss who are at least 18 years old.

John Tracy Clinic
806 W. Adams Blvd.
Los Angeles, CA 90007
800-522-4582 (Voice/TDD)
213-748-5481 (Voice)
213-747-2924 (TDD)
213-749-1651 (Fax)
jtclinic@aol.com (E-mail)
www.johntracyclinic.org (Web site)

Provides world-wide parent-centered services to young children with hearing loss. Offers an on-site educational facility for pre-school-age children, focusing on a spoken language environment for the deaf and hard of hearing; educational materials and publications for parents of deaf children and professionals working with the deaf and hard of hearing; correspondence courses; summer programs; and teacher training programs.

National Association of the Deaf (NAD)
814 Thayer Ave.
Silver Spring, MD 20910-4500
301-587-1788 (Voice)
301-587-1789 (TDD)
301-587-1791 (Fax)
NADHQ@juno.com (E-mail)
www.nad.org (Web site)

A private, nonprofit organization providing grassroots advocacy and empowerment to safeguard the accessibility and civil rights of deaf and hard-of-hearing persons, including education, employment, health care, social services, and telecommunications. Provides captioned media, certification of ASL and Deaf Studies professionals, certification of sign language interpreters, deafness-related information and publications, legal assistance, policy development and research, public awareness, and youth leadership development.

National Association of the Deaf Law Center
301-587-7730
301-587-0234 (Fax)
Legal services and resources.

Junior National Association for the Deaf
juniornad@juno.com (E-Mail)

Develops and promotes citizenship, scholarship, and leadership skills in students who are deaf or hard of hearing (grades 7–12) through chapter projects, national conventions, contests, and other activities. Has a month-long Youth Leadership Camp program each summer in Oregon.

National Captioning Institute
1900 Gallows Rd., Suite 3000
Vienna, VA 22182
703-917-7600 (Voice/TDD)
703-917-9878 (Fax)
www.ncicap.org (Web site)

Captioning service for television networks, program producers, cable-casters, producers of home entertainment videocassettes, advertisers, and other organizations in the federal and private sector.

National Council of State Boards of Examiners for Speech-Language Pathology and Audiology
Ken Gist, Executive Secretary
P.O. Box 326
Wellsburg, WV 26070
304-737-2395
KGist@wvwise.org (E-mail)

Organization that gathers information for state licensing boards across the country and addresses issues pertinent to licensing boards. The Council can refer parents or professionals to their local/ state license boards.

National Cued Speech Association
23970 Hermitage Rd.
Cleveland, OH 44122-4008
800-459-3529 (Voice/TDD)
cuedspdisc@aol.com (E-mail)

www.cuedspeech.org (Web site)

Membership organization that provides advocacy and support regarding the use of cued speech. Information and services are provided for people of all ages who are deaf or hard of hearing, their families and friends, and professionals who work with them.

National Easter Seal Society
230 W. Monroe St., Suite 1800
Chicago, IL 60606-4802
312-726-6200 (Voice)
800-221-4602 (Voice)
312-726-4258 (TDD)
www.easter-seals.org (Web site)

Physical medicine, rehabilitation services, and advocacy to help children and adults with disabilities gain greater independence to achieve their goals. Services for children 0–18 years include home and center-based early intervention for children 0–36 months, child care services, preschool programs for children with special needs, after-school care programs, and services for school-age children. Vocational training and employment services for young people and adults with disabilities are also provided.

National Information Center on Deafness (NICD)
Gallaudet University
800 Florida Ave. NE
Washington, DC 20002-3695
202-651-5051 (Voice)
202-651-5052 (TDD)
202-651-5054 (Fax)

nicd@gallux.gallaudet.edu
(E-mail)
www.gallaudet.edu/~nicd
(Web site)

Centralized source of up-to-date information and publications on topics dealing with deafness and hearing loss. The NICD collects, develops, and disseminates information about all aspects of hearing loss and services offered to deaf and hard of hearing people across the nation. Maintains a Directory of National Organizations of and for Deaf and Hard of Hearing People. Also provides information about Gallaudet University.

National Information Center for Children and Youth with Disabilities (NICHCY)
P.O. Box 1492
Washington, DC 20013-1492
800-695-0285 (Voice/TDD)
202-884-8200 (Voice/TDD)
202-884-8441 (Fax)
nichcy@aed.org (E-Mail)
www.nichcy.org (Web site)

National information and referral clearinghouse that provides information on disabilities and disability-related issues, with a special focus on children birth to age 22. Provides State Resource Sheets and information regarding national organizations. A publications catalog is available.

National Information Clearinghouse on Children Who Are Deaf-Blind (DB-LINK)

DB-LINK
Teaching Research
345 N. Monmouth Ave.
Monmouth, OR 97361
800-438-9376 (Voice)
800-854-7013 (TDD)
503-838-8150 (Fax)
dblink@tr.wou.edu (E-mail)
www.tr.wou.edu/dblink
(Web site)

Federally funded (Department of Education, Office of Special Education) information and referral service that identifies, coordinates, and disseminates information related to children (0–21 years) who are deaf-blind.

National Institute on Deafness and Other Communication Disorders (NIDCD) Information Clearinghouse
One Communication Ave.
Bethesda, MD 20892-3456
800-241-1044 (Voice)
800-241-1055 (TDD)
301-907-8830 (Fax)
nidcd@aerie.com (E-mail)
www.nih.gov/nidcd (Web site)

National information resource center, which also conducts and supports biomedical research and research training, for normal and disordered processes of hearing, balance, smell, taste, voice, speech, and language. The Clearinghouse develops health-related materials, such as directories, information packets, fact sheets, and pamphlets about deafness and communication disorders. It serves health professionals, patients, industry, and the public. NIDCD is one of the Institutes that comprise the National Institutes of Health (NIH), which is part of the U.S. Department of Health and Human Services.

NIDCD Hereditary Hearing Impairment Resource Registry (HHIRR)
Boys Town National Research Hospital
555 N. 30th St.
Omaha, NE 68131
800-320-1171 (Voice/TDD)
402-498-6331 (Fax)
NIDCD_HHIRR@boystown.org (E-mail)

National Neurofibromatosis Foundation, Inc. (NNFF)
95 Pine St., 16th Floor
New York, NY 10005
800-323-7938
NNFF@aol.com (E-mail)

Support of research to find effective treatments and a cure for neurofibromatosis (NF). Direct services, information, and resources are available to children and adults with NF.

National Technical Institute for the Deaf (NTID)
Rochester Institute of Technology
One Lomb Memorial Dr.
P.O. Box 9887
Rochester, NY 14623
716-475-6700 (Voice/TDD)
716-475-6500 (Fax)
www.rit.edu/~418www (Web site)

One of seven colleges of Rochester Institute of Technology (RIT). The world's first and largest technical college for deaf students. Provides technical and professional educational programs for the deaf. NTID also prepares professionals to work in fields related to deaf people, has a program of applied research, and shares its knowledge and expertise through outreach and other programs. Disseminates information and instructional videotapes on issues related to deaf people and deaf culture.

Network for Overcoming Increased Silence Effectively (NOISE)
listserver@lists.acs.ohio-state.edu

Listserver for hard-of-hearing and deaf medical professionals and for professional students with hearing loss (at least age 15) who are interested in a medical career.

New York League for the Hard of Hearing
71 W. 23rd St.
New York, NY 10010-4162
212-741-7650 (Voice)
212-255-1932 (TDD)
212-255-4413 (Fax)
postmaster@lhh.org (E-mail)
www.lhh.org (Web site)

Oldest hearing rehabilitation agency in the country, with a mission to improve the quality of life for people with all degrees of hearing loss. Offers comprehensive hearing rehabilitation and human service programs for infants, children, adults, and their families, regardless of age or mode of communication. Promotes hearing conservation and provides public education about hearing.

San Francisco SPCA Hearing Dog Program
2500 16th St.
San Francisco, CA 94103-6589
415-554-3020 (Voice)
415-554-3022 (TDD)
hearingdog@sfspca.org (E-mail)
www.sfspcahdp.org (Web site)

Hearing dogs are chosen from shelters, trained, and placed with persons 18 years old and over in the states of California and Nevada. (Dogs may be placed with younger persons, considered on a case-by-case basis.) The application fee is $20 and the class fee is $100.

The SEE Center for the Advancement of Deaf Children
P. O. Box 1181
Los Alamitos, CA 90720
562-430-1467 (Voice/TDD)
562-795-6614 (Fax)

Information and referral for parents and educators regarding deafness-related topics and Signing Exact English (SEE). Provides evaluation of signing skills, workshops, and consulting services related to communication in general and SEE in particular.

Self Help for Hard of Hearing People, Inc.
7910 Woodmont Ave., Suite 1200

Bethesda, MD 20814
301-657-2248 (Voice)
301-657-2249 (TDD)
301-913-9413 (Fax)
national@shhh.org (E-mail)
www.shhh.org (Web site)

Nonprofit educational organization dedicated to the welfare and interests of those who cannot hear well and their friends and relatives. Promotes advocacy, self help, awareness, and information about hearing loss, communication, assistive devices, and alternative communication skills through publications, exhibits, and presentations.

Sertoma International/Sertoma Foundation, Inc.
1912 E. Meyer Blvd.
Kansas City, MO 64132-1174
816-333-8300 (Voice/TDD)
www.sertoma.org (Web site)

Service club that emphasizes communication disorders. Provides $1,000 scholarships for students who are deaf or hard of hearing for 4-year Bachelor's Degree. (Send self-addressed, stamped envelope to the address listed to request an application.) Also provides camps for children with communication disorders; "Quiet Pleases" videotape series about speech and hearing, including teacher guides (one of which— "Listen Up! For the Sounds of Your Life!"—is available free from many Blockbuster video stores); and "Johnny Guitar Comix" for 2nd–5th grade children regarding harmful effects of loud noise. Local Sertoma Clubs can request up to $10,000 in matching funds for local speech and hearing projects.

Social Security Administration
Contact local Social Security office or call:
800-772-1213 (Voice)
800-325-0778 (TDD)
www.ssa.gov (Web site)

Information on Social Security programs and benefits, how to apply for benefits, how to reach a local office, and so forth.

Telecommunications for the Deaf, Inc.
8630 Fenton St., Suite 604
Silver Spring, MD 20910-3803
301-589-3786 (Voice)
301-589-3006 (TDD)
301-589-3797 (Fax)
tdiexdir@ad.com (E-mail)
www.tdi-online.org (Web site)

Nonprofit consumer advocacy organization promoting full visual access to entertainment, information, and telecommunications for people who are deaf, hard of hearing, deaf-blind, and speech impaired. Conducts consumer education, technical assistance, application of existing and emerging technologies, networking and collaborations, uniformity of standards, national policy development, and advocacy.

Tele-Consumer Hotline
901 15th St., NW, Suite 230
Washington, DC 20005

800-332-1124 (Voice/TDD/Fax)

Impartial consumer information service about residential telecommunications concerns. Information and referrals about equipment and phone services for consumers with disabilities. Free publications about telephone equipment, TDD directories, relay services, selecting a long-distance company, and so forth.

United States Department of Education
600 Independence Ave., SW
Washington, DC 20202-0498
800-USA-LEARN
CustomerService@inet.ed.gov (E-mail)
www.ed.gov (Web site)

Information regarding programs and services, publications, offices and budgets, student financial assistance, legislation, regulations and policies, and so forth.

Office of Special Education and Rehabilitation Services (OSERS) Communication and Information Services
Switzer Building, Room 3132
330 C St., SW
Washington, DC 20202-2524
202-205-8241
http://inet.ed.gov/~dsti/
OSERS (Web site)

Supports programs that assist in educating children with special needs, provides for the rehabilitation of youth and adults with disabilities, and supports research to improve the lives of individuals with disabilities. Has three components: the Rehabilitation Services Administration (RSA), the National Institute on Disability and Rehabilitative Research (NIDRR), and the Office of Special Education Program (OSEP). The focus of OSEP is on free and appropriate public education of children and youth with disabilities from birth to 21 years. Its major responsibilities involve administering the provisions and programs of the Individuals with Disabilities Education Act (IDEA).

Rehabilitation Services Administration (RSA) Deafness and Communicative Disorders Branch
Switzer Building, Room 3228
330 C St., SW
Washington, DC 20202-2736
202-205-9152 (Voice)
202-205-8352 (TDD)
202-205-9340 (Fax)

Promotes rehabilitation services for people who are deaf or hard of hearing and for individuals with speech-language impairment; technical assistance to public and private organizations and agencies regarding vocational rehabilitation; and funding for interpreter training and demonstration rehabilitation programs.

Venture Clubs of the Americas
Attn: Venture Student Aid Award
Soroptimist International
2 Penn Center Plaza, Suite 1000
Philadelphia, PA 19102-5200
215-557-9300

Student scholarships for 15–40 year olds with physical disabilities and financial need. To receive an application, send a self-addressed, stamped envelope to the address above.

APPENDIX 9–D

BEGINNING HEARING AID USE
(Note: Not all questions may apply to all children.)

Does your child willingly wear the hearing aids?

☐ always: _____

☐ sometimes: _____

☐ not often: _____

☐ never: _____

How easy is it to put on the earmolds and hearing aids?

☐ very easy

☐ easy

☐ difficult

☐ very difficult

Once the earmolds are inserted orrectly and the hearing aids are in place, do the hearing aids whistle?

☐ always: ☐ right   ☐ left

☐ sometimes: ☐ right   ☐ left

☐ not often: ☐ right   ☐ left

☐ never: ☐ right   ☐ left

How easy is it to change the batteries?

☐ very easy

☐ easy

☐ difficult

☐ very difficult

Does your child complain about or show signs of discomfort from the hearing aids or earmolds (e.g., redness, sore ears, etc.)?

☐ always: _____

☐ sometimes: _____

☐ not often: _____

☐ never: _____

Do loud sounds or voices seem annoying?

☐ always: _____

☐ sometimes: _____

☐ not often: _____

☐ never: _____

How well does your child hear in large groups or noisy environments?

☐ very poorly: _____

☐ not very well: _____

☐ pretty well: _____

☐ very well: _____

How well does your child hear in small groups or quiet conversation?

☐ very poorly: _____

☐ not very well: _____

☐ pretty well: _____

☐ very well: _____

Does your child hear soft sounds and voices?

☐ usually: _____

☐ sometimes: _____

☐ not often: _____

☐ never: _____

Does your child hear/understand your voice?

☐ always: _____

☐ most of the time: _____

☐ not often: _____

☐ never: _____

When watching TV or listening to music, how loud is the volume?

☐ too high

☐ too low

☐ normal

Do you have any concerns or questions?

_____

_____

_____

How do you feel about the benefit your child is receiving from the hearing aids?

_____

_____

_____

_____

Day/Date	Length of Time Worn	Responses Observed to Sound
_____	_____	_____
_____	_____	_____
_____	_____	_____
_____	_____	_____
_____	_____	_____
_____	_____	_____
_____	_____	_____
_____	_____	_____
_____	_____	_____
_____	_____	_____

Name of Child: _____

Person Reporting: _____

Make/Model of Hearing Aids: _____

The final chapter in this book deals with "the dark side" of our profession. As stated in the first few chapters, the world is made up of a lot of different personalities (e.g., some good, some bad, some honest, some deceitful). As professionals, we must find a way to deal with all of these types of individuals. Certainly, the vast majority of our patients fit the mold of people who are coming to us for assistance and guidance. Unfortunately, there are a few patients who seem to have been placed on this earth simply to make our jobs difficult (to put it mildly). In the final chapter, Joyce Johnson, Lori Pakulski, and Helena Solodar present a series of such cases and offer helpful strategies on how to provide the best services to these individuals while at the same time guarding the security of our own practices and businesses.

10

Dealing With "Challenging" Patients

■ **Joyce Johnson, M.A.** ■
■ **Lori Pakulski, Ph.D.** ■
■ **Helena Solodar, M.A.** ■

We have all experienced challenging patients, those who feel they deserve *all* of our time, those who require special attention, and those who leave us totally frustrated and fatigued. Although time consuming, we must listen to our patients and hear what they say. Some require patience and tender, gentle guidance, whereas others require a firm hand.

PATIENTS REQUIRING UNDERSTANDING: ILLUSTRATIVE CASES

Less Than Coordinated Patients

Dexterity issues must always be considered when fitting hearing instruments. Patients often want the smallest, least visible products regardless of their manual dexterity, visual acuity, ear size and condition, or hearing loss. In addition to the impact that arthritis or other problems may have on their ability to manipulate the hearing aids, even individuals with no specific medical concerns who have large or clumsy hands may have problems changing batteries, manipulating the instruments, and putting them in their ears.

Case

Mrs. Allthumbs was tested by the audiologist and found to have a moderate, sloping to severe sensorineural hearing loss. She was a diminutive lady who was concerned about her appearance. Her hands were arthritic and she needed a magnifying glass to read. She was concerned about the size of the hearing aids. She wanted to purchase the "invisible" aids advertised on television. But after 90 minutes of trying to insert and remove the batteries and trying to insert the hearing aids in her ears, she agreed to try a larger style.

Tips

- Have sample hearing aids for patients to handle and manipulate. Demonstrate how each style will look in or on the ear.
- Let each patient handle the different battery sizes. Explain that the smaller the hearing aid, the smaller the battery.
- *Before ordering the hearing aids*, insist that the patient demonstrate the ability to manipulate and operate model devices.
- Have the patient manipulate the volume control wheels on each model. If the patient is unable to adjust the volume control wheel, consider a screw set volume control. Another option is a more sophisticated product, such as an instrument that utilizes a remote control or an automatically adjusting hearing aid.
- Remind the patient that ear size must be considered. A small, curvy ear canal will not accommodate a completely-in-the-canal (CIC), and an ear that is close to the head will be difficult to place a behind-the-ear hearing aid on. Often, an ear impression is necessary to determine the best style. Although we are not advocating being untruthful, if you are certain that the patient will fail with certain styles (yet succeed with others), find reasons to dissuade the patient from the improper style. For example, you could "emphasize" certain limitations, such as curvature of the ear canal, that patients can neither verify nor dispute.
- Telephone use with a hearing aid is sometimes improved when a "telephone switch" is added to the hearing aid. Because this small toggle switch can be difficult to feel and move, consider other alternatives such as an amplified telephone, a telephone pad, or similar devices.

- Consider a referral to an occupational therapist (or enlist the help of other team members if a patient is currently in rehabilitation) to help refine motor skills or seek alternative ways to manipulate the necessary components of the hearing aid.
- Consider an assistive listening device rather than a small hearing aid when patients are not able to manipulate anything small and they have no one else to provide assistance.

Perceptually Confused Patients

The aging process brings many changes. One of these changes is confusion or memory loss that may occur gradually or suddenly. Teaching patients who are senile or have Alzheimer's disease to use and care for their hearing aids takes time and an extraordinary amount of patience. Keep in mind that the appearance of patients is not indicative of their mental capabilities.

Case

Mr. Bliss, a long-time hearing aid user, was exhibiting increasing difficulty completing the basic daily use and care of his hearing instruments. His wife now had to drive him to office visits and she complained constantly of his incompetence. Over several months, Mr. Bliss and his wife were seen for short visits nearly once a week. Mr. Bliss would hand over a large cigar box filled with various pieces and parts from a lifetime of hearing aid use and forget to bring along or wear his current hearing aids. When he did have his current instruments, problems included a dead battery, disconnected tubing on his earmold, upside down battery, or the on-off switch in the incorrect position. At each visit, his wife would monopolize the appointment complaining and often berating him for his poor memory. Because Mr. Bliss and his wife traveled a long distance to come to the office, the clinician increasingly sought Mrs. Bliss's assistance to help her husband troubleshoot the devices. Despite this encouragement, she refused, stating that she already had the burden of caring for everything else. With Mrs. Bliss' permission, the clinician enlisted a neighbor who drove down for a visit and received troubleshooting lessons. The kindly neighbor visited Mr. Bliss each day and assisted him in managing the hearing aids and called the office when he had questions.

Eventually, Mr. Bliss worsened and was admitted to the Alzheimer's care center. In-service training was provided to the nursing staff and occasional visits were made to check on Mr. Bliss. Despite his other problems, Mr. Bliss was able to maintain contact to the best of his ability.

Tips

- Have patience with your patients. It is difficult to understand the negative impact of hearing loss on persons and their relationships, especially when it is accompanied by other medical or psychological problems.
- When possible, enlist help from others in the family, circle of friends, or other care providers to provide support for the person with the hearing loss and anyone who is having difficulty dealing with that person.
- Try to provide readable props or instructions with large pictures for daily care of the instruments.
- Allow patients to come in frequently for short visits if possible. Mr. Bliss benefited greatly from appointments that took only a few minutes of professional time. He was grateful and willing (and able) to pay for the help.
- Consider simple Assistive Listening Devices (ALDs) such as a Pocket Talker with a self-contained microphone and earplugs or a headset.
- Make certain that the patient has appropriate extended insurance coverage for loss and damage.

Depressed Patients

Most people want a long life, but few enjoy growing old. Depression is common in the geriatric population. Feelings of abandonment, loneliness, and isolation abound as general health deteriorates.

Case

Mrs. Downer, age 83, complained bitterly about growing old. She routinely told the staff that growing old is hell, and she had not found any gold in her golden years. She reported a long list of ailments and medications. When told that she needed hearing aids, she said "That will be the last nail in my coffin. Everything is falling apart, first my eyes, then my teeth, and now my ears. I may be bad off, but I'm not that far gone that I need hearing aids."

Tips

- Empathize with patients' concerns about aging. Validate their health issues.

- Don't say "I know what you're going through," because you don't. Instead you might say you have seen others going through health issues and you can imagine how difficult that must be.
- Make patients understand that hearing loss occurs in children and young adults too. You might even introduce them to a younger person wearing hearing aids.
- Reassure patients that you will spend time teaching them to use and care for the hearing aids and that eventually the process will take only minutes a day.
- Reiterate that the use of hearing aids can greatly enhance the quality of one's life, mainly by minimizing social isolation.
- Arrange frequent follow-up appointments until the patient is comfortable with the hearing aids.
- Remind patients that hearing aid use is not just to improve hearing. It also allows people to remain more independent, active, and healthier.
- Inform patients that better hearing will make them more desirable socially, and family and friends will find it easier to interact with them.
- Provide information on support groups and organizations such as Self Help for the Hard of Hearing (SHHH).
- Don't force amplification on patients.
- Know when and where to refer for professional mental health assistance.

Patients in Denial

Denial can produce serious complications. The phenomenon is common among people of all ages, affecting males and females. These patients may claim that other people mumble or speak with their backs turned. They might complain that young people today have not been taught to speak properly, and the television announcers and actors are in need of elocution exercises.

Case

Mrs. Noway was brought to the office by her son. She claimed that she was hearing everything she wanted to hear. Her son related instances when she either did not hear or answered questions inappropriately. He tried to tell her that at times she spoke too loudly and that the grandchildren were tired of repeating things to her. After the testing, she was found to have a moderate hearing loss in both ears. The audiologist had the responsibility to convince her of the need for amplification without causing her embarrassment in front of her son.

Tips

■ Be sensitive. Keep in mind that just like the previous case, gradual loss of a sense is scary.

■ Educate patients by using objective data gathered during the evaluation. For example, during the hearing evaluation, assess speech discrimination not only at the usual sensation level, but also at a soft conversational level or in the presence of competing noise. This will provide more leverage when explaining to a patient what he is missing.

■ Following the hearing evaluation, provide a thorough and understandable explanation of the findings. Do this by describing what it is that you know the patient will hear and how it will be easy for him to misunderstand because of the nature and degree of the loss. Acknowledging that he really does hear most speech, but that he will miss the important, softer sounds that help to distinguish words, may provide him with a face saving explanation about why he claims he can hear adequately now. Further, illustrate how he might get by in a one-on-one situation but has greater difficulty in a group.

■ Describe the slow but steady progression of hearing loss and how this affects a patient's ability to notice the change. Use an example such as the following: "Persons living next to a railroad track will often not notice that loud trains go by all times of the day and night. They just get used to the sound. When we lose our hearing, it has a similar effect. Typically, we get used to an increasingly quiet world. Soon, we do not realize how much we are missing."

■ Enlist a trusted family member to encourage (but not force) patients to try amplification.

■ Enlist a trusted physician, if necessary, who may have persuasive powers that you have not yet been granted with the patient. Be sure to provide the physician with a thorough description of the nature of the loss and the possible benefits of amplification.

■ Discuss the changes in lifestyle that may have occurred (or may be at the brink of occurring) due to the person's inability to communicate effectively.

■ Discuss the significance of the trial or adjustment period. Convince patients that they will make their family (and/or friends) happy if they just give the hearing aids a try. ("Do it for others, if not for yourself.") Then, patients will have the control to determine if there is improvement with hearing aids.

■ Send patients a written follow-up explaining the audiologic results and the significance of those findings in relation to conversational level speech. In the report, include information related to possible benefits of amplification.

PATIENTS REQUIRING A FIRM HAND: ILLUSTRATIVE CASES

"Walk-In" Patients

The problems with walk-ins are universal to the hearing health care profession, regardless if you work in a private clinic, university clinic, or hospital. Walk-in patients can be extremely disruptive. If you "work in" the patient, you run the risk of delaying a scheduled patient, or if you make the walk-in patient wait, scheduled patients in the waiting area observing the situation may misinterpret that you are mistreating an apparently nice patient.

Case

Mr. Walken is a patient with a profound hearing loss who has been coming to the clinic for years. He uses behind-the-ear hearing aids with limited benefit and relies heavily on speechreading to understand speech. He uses gestures but has chosen not to learn any formal sign language. In addition to the hearing loss, there are also some apparent cognitive deficits. Mr. Walken can read some basic phrases and is employed at a program that allows for his special needs.

When Mr. Walken is in need of audiological assistance, he comes to the clinic and sits and quietly waits until someone is available to see him. He has been known to wait several hours. If an audiologist is not available, the receptionist will make an appointment, comparing calendars and completing an appointment card. However, this is fruitless, because Mr. Walken rarely keeps the appointed time. Instead he will return another day, without an appointment, and sit and wait quietly for someone to assist him.

Not all walk-in patients are as pleasant as Mr. Walken. In fact, many walk-in patients can be impatient and even abusive, demanding immediate attention. It is difficult to settle this situation, whether the walk-in person is undemanding or rude.

Tips

■ Let the receptionist handle all walk-ins. This will prevent the audiology staff from spending valuable time explaining why they are unavailable at the moment. The reception staff should begin by asking patients if they have an appointment, thereby reminding them of appropriate office protocol. Second, inform patients that the audiologists' schedules will be checked to see if they can be worked in. Another option, depending on the patients' needs, would include asking them to leave the hearing aid for someone to check at a later time. Assure patients that you will follow up with a phone call. Or, ask walk-in patients to make an appointment at a convenient time for them to return when the audiologist would be available to address their needs.

■ Document, document, document. Always note in patients' records that they were walk-ins and note occasions when they were seen without an appointment. If a person is a repeat walk-in, it might prove beneficial to put a colored sticker on the outside of the chart to remind you at a glance.

■ When the audiologist is able to see "walk-in" patients, begin by firmly (but kindly) reiterating the need and importance of an appointment. Briefly describe how tightly patients are scheduled and that an appointment time will prevent previously scheduled people as well as "walk-ins" from being inconvenienced by having to wait or return at another time. Also, remind them that the mission of your office is to provide the best possible care. To do so, you need appropriate time to prepare for patients, work with them, and arrange any necessary follow-up. Tell them that, certainly, they can understand and appreciate this concept.

■ Consider whether it may be cost efficient to hire a technical assistant to address the needs and concerns of walk-ins. Remind walk-in patients that they will always see the technician, not the audiologist. You may even consider charging higher fees for walk-ins.

Professional Patients

Professionals, particularly those in the health care field, can present dilemmas as patients. Because they may also be referral sources, there can be an expectation that you will return favors by meeting their special needs or providing substantial discounts. Further, in light of their demanding schedules, there might be an expectation that you will accommodate them as necessary. Hearing is paramount to the services they provide, thus high demands are created regarding hasty completion of repairs and immediate rendering of services.

Case

Dr. Godley had a long-standing progressive sensorineural hearing loss. Although Dr. Godley had been aware of this loss for a long time, he had chosen not to wear amplification or seek medical advice. In the latter part of his education, Dr. Godley became increasingly aware of missed information due to the loss of hearing. When he finally decided to seek a consultation regarding these concerns, he stated that he must have the smallest (invisible) hearing aid or surgery to correct the problem because he was concerned about being discriminated against because of his hearing loss.

Dr. Godley was tested, counseled, and impressions were taken for completely-in-the-canal hearing aids with a description of the possible fitting problems because of the borderline candidacy with his hearing loss and his small, sensitive ear canals. In addition, he was advised to seek further medical consultation beyond the medical clearance he had received from a colleague to investigate the nature and cause of the progressive loss.

Documentation of subsequent visits shows that Dr. Godley returned over several years nearly a hundred times, during which he experienced continued fitting problems, significant decrease in hearing, and wax-related concerns. He refused to believe that his hearing was diminishing, but blamed worsening test results on tinnitus, stress, and fatigue. He refused to try instruments other than CICs, despite his inability to hear well in many situations. And, the documents are peppered with comments of both admonishment and praise for services and time frames in which those services were rendered. Further, he often balked at charges because he believed it was the audiologist's obligation to "make things right" without taking ownership of any of the problems he was experiencing.

Tips

■ Begin by inquiring about and documenting patients' needs and expectations. Thoughtfully, but forcefully, inform patients about ways in which your office may or may not be able to meet their expectations. Offer to refer for additional assistance if necessary.

■ Carefully explain necessary procedures and the reasons for them. For example, if there is a question about why it takes a week to get a hearing aid repaired, remind patients that the manufacturer is in another state and therefore, there may be limitations in delivery and benchwork time (particularly over weekends).

- Encourage these patients to purchase two sets of hearing aids. This will provide them with spare instruments so that they are not left without hearing aids during an important work day or meeting.
- Offer them the option of getting a second opinion from a colleague.

Know-It-All Patients

Many patients have some degree of expertise in audiology or in a related area. Occasionally, these individuals feel the need to educate you, the professional who will be managing their hearing health care needs. At other times, persons with "know-it-all" attitudes may challenge or question your knowledge and authority.

Case

Mr. Wright, a retired engineer, had visited many clinics and tried several hearing aids before making an appointment at our office. He reported that the hearing aids he had tried before did not meet his expectations. "If we are able to put a man on the moon, we should be able to restore hearing to near perfect without constant breakdowns and problems," he would say. Further, he expected an in-depth explanation of all components, available technology, and then questioned why audiologists have not completed degrees in electronics or engineering.

Tips

- Compliment patients on their knowledge. Mention that it is enjoyable for you to be able to discuss technical issues.
- Educate patients regarding differences between their areas of expertise and yours. "I may not be an engineer, but I know how hearing aids work and what limitations there are based on the integrity of the auditory system."
- Before discussing hearing aids, talk about the hearing loss from the standpoint of what the patient is missing. This will confirm that you do have some understanding of his needs. Discuss technical limitations of hearing aids in conjunction with the patient's impaired auditory system.
- For technically oriented patients who question why hearing aids cannot correct impaired hearing when scientists have "landed people on the moon," explain complexities of the auditory system including impaired sensitivity, abnormal loudness perception, frequency selectivity, temporal integration, and localization ability.

- Provide patients with as detailed an explanation as appropriate and use documents and test results that fulfill their desires to be informed. This may also build confidence in the sophistication and expertise that is involved in the entire process. Previously prepared technical papers, manufacturer specifications, and real ear results may provide valuable examples.
- Within reason, ask for patients' input regarding technological aspects that might interest or frustrate them the most. Further, letting patients know that you are communicating with the manufacturer may also prove beneficial.
- If patients appear likely to modify the instrument or explore the internal components, caution them that certain changes may affect the warranty status.
- If patients feel they can make adjustments for themselves, remind them that knowledge of the hearing aid circuitry and specifications may not suffice. However, if the particular system allows for it, give them a chance. If this necessitates further adjustments by you, let them know there will be a charge for your services.
- Remind patients that hearing aid fidelity is limited by the fact that they are powered by a 1.4 volt battery.
- Document, document, document. It is important to document objectives, discussions, and materials you have provided for future reference. Also critical is that you document hearing aid settings and hearing aid integrity. If you get a "tinkerer," you want proof if the patient adjusted the hearing aid settings or modified the instrument in some other way, especially if it might affect the manufacturer's warranty.
- Do not engage in a "contest" of who knows more.
- Do not give in to bullying. If a patient continues to question or berate your abilities, remind him that he may not wish to continue paying you for such services.

Dishonest Patients

Unfortunately, there are dishonest people in the world, and some may also be dishonest patients who can be damaging to the practice and the staff. Dishonest patients may lie about services received, staff treatment, or satisfaction level. Further, their stories may change over time. If other patients are privy to their stories, those patients can become wary about your services. Sometimes, dishonest patients may inform the audiologist that the office staff is incompetent or behaves improperly. Chronic liars may try to tell the office staff that the audiologist promised certain things to them. Other times, the destructive behaviors may be exhibited in working one audiologist against another.

Case

Mrs. Lyon was a 76-year-old female with a moderate hearing loss. She was fit with binaural, programmable hearing aids. When scheduling her 2-week check, Mrs. Lyon asked to see a more experienced audiologist. Her complaints ranged from not being given a thorough test to being promised a discount that was not honored. At her next visit, she requested an extension of her trial program, stating that she was not given sufficient information on the use and care of the instrument and subsequently was not prepared to make a decision about keeping the hearing aids. At her final trial period appointment, she requested a third audiologist. She reported that the previous audiologist was rude and abusive. Approximately 6 months later, Mrs. Lyon returned to get the hearing aids replaced because she had never been satisfied with them (despite documented reports of success at each visit). When she was told that she could not return the hearing aids because of the completion of the trial period, she became irate stating that she had not been informed of a trial period (despite the fact that she had signed a contract).

Tips

- Maintain consistency among all staff members in office policies and procedures.
- Create checklists that can be reviewed with all patients to establish what services are recommended and have been received, including costs for those services, policies and procedures for services ranging from caring for hearing aids, using the instruments, battery safety, warranty, and follow-up.
- Always schedule a set time frame for each procedure so that patients cannot claim favoritism or special treatment by certain professionals.
- Maintain a written price schedule including information about insurance reimbursement. If there is a discount or special, include that offer and the particulars about it. Ask patients to sign and date it, place a copy in the chart, and give a copy to them for future reference.
- Provide every patient with an appointment card, written in ink, and give a copy to a family member or friend if someone accompanies the patient. (If the case is difficult, make a copy and place that in the chart as well.)
- Do not listen to complaints or concerns about staff without another staff member present. This will show honest patients that you are taking their concerns seriously. If a patient is dishonest, it puts him in an uncomfortable position of having a second person to dispute

problems. If appropriate, bring the "accused" staff in and ask the patient to address the problems face-to-face.
■ Document, document, document.

Thieving Patients

Health care, like any other business, is susceptible to fraud. When hearing aids are dispensed and services rendered, much cost is involved. Thieves may come in sheep's clothing: an aged "grandma" figure or a business executive. Sometimes, the payments are in the form of bad checks. Other times, there may be a cancellation of insurance with no means of recovering your costs.

Case

Mr. Steele was referred to the clinic for a trial with amplification by his physician. At his first visit, he completed a case history that included new patient information such as address, employer, and insurance information. He stated that he was entitled to two hearing aids through his insurance company. Later he was fit with binaural hearing aids. He returned for his 2-week appointment stating that he was quite satisfied. When he missed his postfitting appointment, a phone call was made to remind him. Because there was no answer, a note was sent in the mail. His insurance company was billed. A few weeks later, the letter was returned with no forwarding address, and the insurance company sent a denial stating that Mr. Steele no longer had insurance coverage. When his employer was called, he reported that Mr. Steele had not worked there in 3 months. Additional calls to his home revealed that he no longer lived at that address and the phone was disconnected.

Tips

■ On the patient intake form, request information about another relative or person not living with the patient.
■ Ask for a daytime phone number of patients or their spouse.
■ Request the patient's social security number.
■ Post or provide a statement reminding patients that passing bad checks is a felony and lack of payment is grand theft. Include information about the availability of reasonable payment schedules.
■ Take the time to verify any insurance coverage before ordering the instruments. Keep copies of patients' insurance cards in their charts. Obtain all relevant insurance data including time frame of coverage, insurance agent's name and phone number, and reimbursable

amount. Have patients sign a form indicating they are responsible for any uninsured fees.

Time-Wasting Patients

At times, patients have needs that call for much greater time and attention than is appropriate or necessary for hearing health care alone. Patients who require excessive time may just like to talk, may need attention, or have vague complaints they want addressed. Many of these patients also fit into the category of "walk-ins," which makes them "double-trouble." The patients may be pleasant and kind or difficult and unruly; all of these traits may require techniques to avoid consumption of valuable time by both the audiologist and the office staff. Keep in mind that patients do not need to be in the office to be using your time in an inappropriate manner. Sometimes, patients who exhibit these behaviors will phone frequently asking for advice, requesting unrelated information, or inquiring about services. Other times, they might request specific information, only to discard that idea as soon as the information is received to move on to a new whim.

Case

Every day was a new day with complaints and problems for Mrs. Weiner. First, she complained of pain in her ear. When this was addressed, she described every encounter with background noise and requested that her hearing aids be adjusted "just a little." That discussion was followed by problems with hearing in groups, battery life concerns, and wax related issues. Each time one problem was resolved, four more arose.

Tips

- Train the receptionist or telephone staff to field questions effectively, "Sir, is your hearing aid not working? We will set up an appointment for you."
- When counseling these patients, avoid discussions on topics not directly related. If patients get off the subject, gently but quickly steer them back.
- Consider office charges for out-of-warranty visits, and inform patients of the number of complimentary visits. Often, patients who are seeking company may avoid an office visit if they are being charged.
- Suggest the Self Help for the Hard of Hearing (SHHH) or a similar group if individuals appear to desire support and friendship.

- Today's technology can encourage a chronic time-waster with different program combinations and options. It may be advisable to present only a few options that provide a sufficient range of choices.
- Isolate overly talkative patients when they arrive so that they cannot continually engage the office staff in conversation while waiting their turn.

Condescending Patients

Some patients seem to have multiple personalities. One staff member might mention that a particular patient is terribly difficult and another audiologist looks at her as if she has lost her mind. These patients may be rude, obnoxious, belligerent, aggressive, and often downright nasty to one person (often the receptionist or technician), but incredibly sweet to another person in the same office. This is not the same as patients who are having a bad day. We have all tolerated patients' needs to "vent" occasionally. The type of patient discussed here is a chronic offender.

Case

Mrs. Snooty was a 70-year-old socialite well known in the community for her parties, fund-raisers, and philanthropic deeds. Her attitude appeared to be one of such self-importance that she deserved to be served by "only the best" or the senior staff member. She was often cold and condescending to all others and immediately transformed into a warm laughing "friend" when with the "boss."

Tips

- "Kill them with kindness." Encourage all staff members to greet these patients with a smile and compliment them because someone of this character may respond well to attention.
- Remember that, because of their status in the community, the way you handle these individuals may influence the success of your practice.
- Praise your staff in front of patients. Remind patients that all members of the staff are valued and trusted.
- Under no circumstances should abusive language be permitted. If necessary, move the offender to a private room. When comfortable, the "senior audiologist" should politely "lay out the rules of conduct" to the offender.

Impatient Patients

Occasionally a person will arrive at the office saying, "I am leaving on a trip overseas in 2 weeks and I want to get hearing aids so that I will be able to enjoy the trip." Although such persons have had hearing loss for the past several years, they typically wait until some critical occasion such as a trip, a wedding, or a big meeting. Then, they want the instruments instantly. A quote from an anonymous author best describes this problem, "A hearing aid is something people wait years to buy and then cannot live without for one day." Even if testing and fitting can occur in the time allowed, there can be additional concerns of hearing aid use under such circumstances without a proper trial period.

Case

Mr. Rush made an appointment 2 days in advance for a hearing test. At the visit, he described himself as an important businessman who frequently travels overseas for long periods. He was scheduled to leave the following week for Japan. He reported a noticeable change in hearing over the past several years and decided it was time to do something about it. He was especially concerned about hearing critical business at his next meeting. He requested that the hearing test and hearing aid fitting be completed before he left.

When we explained the medical clearance process, orientation, and trial program, he wanted a way around it. He replied that he would choose to avoid all of those things, he would take responsibility, and pay whatever price necessary. Knowing he would go elsewhere, our office decided to do the best we could to accommodate him. The medical clearance was faxed that day, the order shipped out overnight with a "rush," and he was fit the day he left for Japan. He was counseled regarding the problems that may arise and so forth. He returned 4 weeks later with a sore ear and some general occlusion problems. He stated that he would be leaving 3 days later for another business trip and needed a fast turn around on the modifications. The demands continued.

Tips

- Educate, educate, educate. Explain the custom-fitting nature of hearing aids and the importance of appropriate fitting time.
- Insist on a 30-day trial period with patients being accessible to the audiologist at least 2 weeks of that time. Remind them that this is in *their* best interest.

- If patients visit another area frequently (such as people who winter in Florida and summer in Michigan), refer them to another respected audiologist in the other place of residence.
- Charge extra for *every* rush order, including the cost of inconvenience to the staff.
- Provide a loaner or assistive listening device until there is time for a custom fit.
- Have written policies you can show to patients.

Careless Patients

Some patients tend to misplace or lose an inordinate number of hearing aids. This may be caused by carelessness, age-related memory problems, or just general irresponsibility. Regardless of the reason, the dispensing audiologist is often faced with having to provide considerable resources, often without reimbursement, to obtain replacements (or loaners) for these patients.

Case

Miss Place, a kind and trustworthy woman, was quite pleased with her new CIC hearing aids at the orientation. She was provided with information on use, care, and specific warranty information for repair, loss, and damage. When she returned in 1 week, she reported that she had lost the hearing aids. New impressions were taken and another set of hearing aids was ordered under the manufacturer's loss and damage warranty. At the following visit, Miss Place was informed of the importance of insurance, should she lose her hearing aids again. Although she stated that she was certain this would not happen again, she did contact her homeowners' insurance and purchased a policy. Two weeks after receiving the second pair, she sheepishly returned to the office to indicate that she had lost another hearing aid. Within 2 months of that incident, Miss Place had a fourth hearing aid eaten by her dog.

Tips

- Always obtain signed documents that information was provided on warranty and insurance. Encourage patients to check with their homeowners' insurance to determine whether coverage is available. These policies are often less expensive and may pay complete replacement costs.
- Provide a large case to store the instruments and a logical method for caring for the hearing aids. Tell patients that when the hearing aids

are not in their ears, they must be stored in the hard case out of reach of any children or animals. A soft case is for use only while getting a hair cut, and so forth, and should not be placed in pockets because the clothing items often end up in the washing machine before the hearing aids are put back in the ears.

■ Charge a replacement fee that is sufficiently high to encourage finding lost hearing aids or deter fraud.

■ Provide a warning about pet damage. Dogs and cats eat hearing aids!

■ For first time offenders, remind them that accidental misplacing of small items happens to many people, not just those who are careless and neglectful.

Angry Patients

Occasionally, patients are angry or irate. An angry patient can be someone who has experienced a bad day or someone who is chronically angry. Patients may be angry because they believe that they have received inappropriate service or they may be unhappy with their hearing aids. Sometimes, angry patients are simply unhappy about everything.

Case

Mr. Tyson ordered a new set of digitally programmable hearing aids. He indicated that he wanted to get the "best" technology. However, his expectations were such that he anticipated a successful adjustment within 2 weeks and believed he would be able to hear perfectly well as soon as he had the devices in. Unfortunately, the laboratory lost his ear impressions and called to request that they be remade. The patient returned to the office for a new set of impressions. The order was rushed, and several days later the hearing aids arrived. Mr. Tyson was fit with the new hearing aids but they were ill fitting. The ear impressions were again taken and sent for remake.

Once again, the new set of hearing aids arrived, and Mr. Tyson was scheduled as soon as schedules permitted. This time the fit was good but feedback was present. After numerous remakes and programming, Mr. Tyson was an angry, disgruntled patient. He complained that for the cost of these instruments, he should not have experienced any of these problems.

Tips

■ Inform patients that hearing aids are made from earmold impressions that must be taken in the office and sent to the manufacturer.

Let them know that the hearing aid fitting is a process and not a single event. Fitting problems arise and hearing aids may need modifications for fitting and acoustic response.

- Prepare patients for the possibility of remakes and that they may not be able to take the hearing aids home after their first visit.
- Provide patients with as much "proof" as possible when there is a shipping or related problem so that they can see it was not the incompetence of the office staff.
- Keep patients well informed. You can diffuse a lot of problems by calling patients and informing them of a problem rather than having them call to check the status only to find out there is a problem.
- "Disarm" the patients' anger by identifying areas of common agreement. It is hard for patients to maintain anger if you agree with them. Then, quickly move on to proposed solutions.

Paranoid Patients

Some patients are concerned that everyone who dispenses hearing aids is a crooked salesman. These patients come into the office after making an appointment giving only their first name to the receptionist on the phone. They saw an advertisement in the paper and are seeking information about a new technology. However, they are concerned that the office will try to trick them into buying something or hassle them afterwards.

Case

When Mr. Nixon arrived for his appointment he refused to sign in or complete a new patient information form. Although he was informed of the office policy, he felt strongly against giving out this information. The audiologist agreed to see him nevertheless. On meeting the audiologist, he immediately informed her that he was there *only* for the *free* hearing screening and information about the new technology. Although he agreed to a demonstration, he constantly reminded the staff that he was not planning to buy hearing aids.

Tips

- With proper training, the office staff can often determine if patients should be scheduled for an appointment or sent information.
- Remind patients that you do not necessarily expect them to make a final decision regarding a hearing aid purchase that day.

■ Try to understand that these individuals have obviously had bad experiences in the past and are overly cautious for a reason. Do not take it personally.

OTHER STRATEGIES

When to "Cut Your Losses"

There will be a few patients in any practice who just are not worth keeping. After much care, a lot of counseling, and a great deal of psychology, you sometimes have to recognize that the patient-clinician relationship is irreparably damaged, and it is time to "call it quits." The following are examples of patients you may want to not treat.

■ Threatening patients. Anyone who threatens you or your staff with bodily harm. No one should have to work under these circumstances.
■ Litigious patients. If patients tell you they have sued an audiologist before or they will sue you if they are not happy, it is best to not treat them.
■ Dissatisfied patients. A patient who is not happy after multiple trials and hours of counseling is one who is not likely to make you happy in the long run.

Tips

■ If you are in a multiple-audiologist practice, determine if you can better meet particular patients' needs by referring them to a colleague. This is best done by calmly and pleasantly asking patients if they would prefer to work with one of your colleagues, explaining a particular virtue possessed by your partner that may benefit them. Further, assure patients that there will be no hard feelings and this is a frequently used professional strategy to ensure that all patients receive the best services possible.
■ If individuals are those you simply do not want as patients, politely inform them that you have exhausted your "bag of tricks." Indicate that you are still interested in assisting them in meeting their needs by directing them to one or more reputable practices. Offer to forward records and part on the best terms possible.

Controlling Your Temper

One of the key factors in controlling anger is to remember that adverse patient behavior is not a personal affront to you. As a consumer, you do not always like every professional with whom you come in contact. Nor do you find that each professional can meet all of your needs. Instead, look on each consumer as an individual whose personal needs and concerns should be addressed by a professional who is able to provide the best services in a way that is pleasing to that patient.

The best defense against difficult patients is a good offense. And that good offense is provided in the form of overt notification of written practice policies. The ground rules must be fair and consistent within the practice. If the rules are established early, it is merely up to the professional to enforce the rules in an appropriate and professional manner. In keeping with this plan, the audiologist must not become emotionally immersed in the dispute or problem. Further, remember that there can be many reasons for a person's actions on a particular day, so do not fall into labeling a patient, but instead deal case by case. By remaining calm and collected, you will maintain control and will more effectively diffuse and resolve problems. Finally, for all "challenging" patients:

- Clarify disagreements rather than arguing. Many disagreements are based on a misunderstanding, so be certain you understand each other.
- Be polite and courteous.
- Discuss the issues; do not attack the patient.
- If you have a disagreement, discuss it in private.
- Propose workable solutions rather than criticizing.

SUMMARY

In dealing with difficult patients, there are a few strategies that can minimize problems.

- Document everything thoroughly. A little extra effort can prevent or diminish future problems.
- Follow-up on potential problems before patients have to call them to your attention. Although it is often preferable to adopt a "wait and see attitude," in the long run problems can be diminished and often avoided if you catch them early.
- Avoid expressing your "feelings." Instead, present every patient with your professionalism.
- Treat them with kindness. Most problems can be avoided if the problem is confronted.
- Stay within your realm of expertise. Do not try to be a psychologist or medical doctor.

And so we have reached the end of our journey. Our goal as hearing health care professionals is to provide patients with the best opportunity to maximize their hearing potential. Hearing aids comprise one piece of that puzzle. If we don't get our patients to wear them, our ability to complete the puzzle is greatly diminished. Despite technological advances, hearing aids remain imperfect. To allow patients to derive the best use of these devices, they must understand the important role of amplification in the larger scope of audiologic rehabilitation. This knowledge can only be conveyed through proper counseling strategies. As professionals, we must become excellent communicators, and that means listening as well as speaking. Never lose sight of the fact that we are in a rehabilitation profession. Even if amplification is initially rejected, the knowledge we convey as counselors can remain invaluable to the well-being of our patients. This handbook contains countless strategies to augment that process. I sincerely hope that you will find them as useful in your practice as I have in mine.

Robert W. Sweetow

I

Index